Managing Ethically

An Executive's Guide

Managing Ethically

An Executive's Guide

Edited by Paul B. Hofmann
and William A. Nelson

HEALTH ADMINISTRATION PRESS

Copyright © 2001 by the Foundation of the American College of Healthcare Executives. Printed in the United States of America. All rights reserved. This book or parts thereof may not be reproduced in any form without written permission of the publisher.

05 04 03 02 01   5 4 3 2 1

Library of Congress Cataloging-in-Publication Data

Hofmann, Paul B., 1941–
    Managing ethically: an executive's guide/Paul B. Hofmann and William A. Nelson.
        p. cm.
    Includes bibliographical references and index.
    ISBN 1-56793-149-9 (alk. paper)
    1. Health services administrators. 2. Medical ethics. 3. Health maintenance organizations—Moral and ethical aspects. I. Nelson, Bill (William A.) II. Title.

        R725.5 .H57 2001
        174'.2—dc21   2001016768
                                                                           CIP

The paper used in this publication meets the minimum requirements of American National Standard for Information Sciences-Permanence of Paper for Printed Library Materials, ANSI Z39.48-1984.♾ ™

Project manager/Editor: Jane Williams; Cover design: Christina Trinidad-Bulla

Health Administration Press
A division of the Foundation of the
    American College of Healthcare Executives
1 North Franklin Street, Suite 1700
Chicago, IL 60606-3491
(312) 424-2800

TABLE OF CONTENTS

PART III   MANAGED CARE

PART IV   MERGERS AND INTEGRATION

PART V   USE OF INFORMATION

PART VI   HUMAN RESOURCES

PART VII   CLINICAL ETHICS ISSUES

PART VIII   ORGANIZATIONAL ETHICS ISSUES

PART IX   INSTITUTIONAL RESOURCES

Introduction

IN 1992 *HEALTHCARE EXECUTIVE* began publishing a regular feature exploring ethical issues under the title, "Healthcare Management Ethics." During the ensuing years, over 50 columns were written by numerous authors. The authors represented a variety of backgrounds, including administrators, scholars, teachers, and ethicists. Despite their professional diversity, they shared a common commitment, along with the American College of Healthcare Executives (ACHE), to foster the development of both ethical leaders and ethical healthcare organizations.

The columns are noteworthy for a variety of reasons. They reflect the wide range of ethical issues encountered by healthcare executives, physicians, employees, patients, and communities. Predictably, clinical concerns have dominated the examination of ethical topics in healthcare since the 1960s. Until relatively recently, the focus was almost exclusively on dilemmas involving individual patients. Allocation of scarce resources, end-of-life decision making, informed consent, abortion, human reproductive technologies, organ transplantation, and similar issues received extensive attention. Despite the appropriate attention devoted to these topics in the general healthcare literature, most healthcare executives deferred to clinicians to resolve them. Nonetheless, executives cannot abdicate responsibility for ensuring that institutional policies and procedures promote patient rights. This obligation is highlighted in a number of the columns.

The columns appropriately expanded the scope of issues beyond a clinical focus to organizational ethics. The authors recognized that dilemmas affecting specific patients should be considered within an institutional context, invariably influenced by the organization's vision, mission, and values. From the beginning, the authors also emphasized how the executive's moral character and integrity have a profound effect on the organization's ethical conscience.

Since the initial publication of these columns, readers have been informed of how the efforts of legislators, the courts, healthcare professionals, ethicists, and the Joint Commission on Accreditation of Healthcare Organizations have contributed to a consensus on a number of critical issues. For example, we endorse the concept that legally competent patients can accept and refuse treatment based on a formal consent-and-refusal process. Furthermore, we confirm that truth-telling and full disclosure should be the norm, and we agree that healthcare ethics committees are a useful resource for developing institutional policies, performing case consultations, and arranging educational programs.

However, just as the columns have expanded the horizon to include both clinical and organizational issues and have identified areas of consensus, they have also examined areas of continued uncertainty. The ethical challenges inherent in supporting managed care, avoiding conflicts of interest and abuse of power, accommodating mergers and acquisitions, and dealing with downsizing are only some of the vexing problems that have no universally accepted solutions.

In addition, the columns acknowledge that ethical discourse should not be left to trained academic ethicists or even the healthcare facility's ethics committee. Ethical reflection is a process that should bring together the values and perspectives of many voices. The columns encourage such a dialogue. Their contents rarely give absolute answers but provide a guide for exploring dilemmas. Such a process leads to ethical discourse, which can bring us closer to acceptable standards of ethical practice.

The ethics columns convey the implicit message that issues are not limited to headline cases highlighting an end-of-life controversy or exposing a failed hospital merger; the columns explore ethical conflicts in the everyday life of executives and their organizations. Depending on how each conflict is addressed, the response either can foster an ethical organization or can erode the ethical culture of the organization. As a result of discussing ethics from an everyday perspective, we can see the importance of integrating ethics discourse into the culture of the organization. The ethics columns promote this objective.

Ethics is not the sole territory of the institution's ethics committee or the compliance office. No group or individual should have exclusive responsibility to serve as the corporate conscience. An ethical organization is achieved not only by having well-crafted policies and procedures, it is achieved when the leadership and entire staff acknowledge the importance of ethical thinking and behavior in the routine and ordinary life of the organization (for example, see Appendix B1 "Health Information Confidentiality"). The ethics columns speak to both patient care concerns and to the manner in which executives treat their staff and relate to the broader community. How is ethics integrated into the fabric of the organization? The very first healthcare management ethics column (by Frankie Perry) urged healthcare executives to "pay even more attention to corporate and personal ethics standards and take the lead to incorporate ethics into the day-to-day activities."

Ethics is not a luxury. It is crucial to the well-being of the organization. The Joint Commission formally acknowledged this point when the first standards on patient rights and organizational ethics were published in 1992. Ethics cannot be left to chance; an ethical organization will not just somehow evolve. An ethical organization is the result of ethical leadership, continuous reflection and planning, ongoing monitoring, and accessible ethics resources (see Appendix B2 "Ethical Decision Making for Healthcare Executives"). Every institution encounters ethical conflicts. The imperative is to recognize them; consider how they should be evaluated within the context of the organization's vision, mission, and values; engage the principal parties in an appropriate decision-making process; and seek ways to prevent such conflicts in the future.

Because the columns are both relevant and practical, they can serve as a useful resource for healthcare executives. With this goal in view, we have compiled the best of the columns originally published in the ethics feature of *Healthcare Executive* magazine. Each column is set apart as its own chapter; the general headings should help the reader locate topics of particular interest. Although this book will not address every ethical conflict encountered by the healthcare executive, it does cover many of the common and familiar issues. In reading the authors' commentaries, you should consider both their perspectives and their reasoning. Ethics reflection is not just a recitation of the answer or a range of appropriate answers; ethics reflection is understanding how to engage in ethical reasoning. In considering the process of "getting there," the reader can review, reflect, and develop ethical skills that can be applied to other conflicts and thus come closer to the goal of being an ethical leader.

The book can be used in a variety ways. All the chapters can be read sequentially, providing the reader with insights into a wide range of ethical conflicts. Alternatively, the reader can review a particular section or chapter that pertains to a current conflict. Instead of reading through an entire chapter, you may want to consider reading the stated ethical conflict or question, pause to think about how you would respond to the conflict, and then read the commentary. Such an approach compares your ethical reasoning with that of the author. Whatever method or format is used, thoughtfully reflecting on the various ethical perspectives will enhance your awareness of ethical issues as well as competing perspectives and values and will provide insights into how executives and organizational policy might address ethical conflicts. In addition to fostering the self-education of executives seeking to enhance their knowledge and skills in ethics, this book can serve as an educational resource for a course, seminar, or ethics discussion group.

The book also contains extensive resource material that will be useful to the healthcare executive. The appendices were specifically developed to provide both the experienced professional and the novice with useful reference documents from ACHE and other sources. ACHE has produced a variety of documents that are intended to guide the ethical behavior of its members.

- The *Code of Ethics* is reviewed and evaluated annually, and it contains standards of ethical behavior for healthcare executives in their professional relationships (see Appendix A).
- The Ethical Policy Statements present ACHE's position on various ethical issues in healthcare and provide advice for executives facing these challenges (see Appendix B1–6).
- The Ethics Self-Assessment Instrument is designed to help executives identify areas of ethical strength and opportunities for further reflection (see Appendix C).

A number of prominent journals serve the field. Although only journals published in the United States are included in Appendix D (Ethics Resources), excellent articles by authors from other countries are published by some of these journals.

Web sites related to ethics continue to proliferate. A list of these web sites is also included in Appendix D.

Most healthcare ethics organizations are part of academic institutions, but some important ones, like The Hastings Center and the Midwest Bioethics Center, are not. Appendix D includes a list of representative ethics institutes, programs, centers, and societies.

A selected bibliography has been included to indicate the impressive array of articles and books on healthcare ethics. This list certainly does not encompass all the relevant publications, but it is a representative sampling of authors and topics worth consideration.

We want to express our appreciation to the many authors who contributed to this book.* Without their effort, this book and *Healthcare Executive's* ethics feature would not exist. We also want to acknowledge the leadership of ACHE and the editors of *Healthcare Executive* for their support. We particularly want to thank Ellen Lanser for serving as our guide in moving forward with this project. In addition, both of us are deeply grateful to the many healthcare executives and managers from whom we have learned over years. Each one has contributed to our growth by raising questions, sharing experiences, identifying uncertainties, and developing creative strategies to help build ethical healthcare organizations.

Paul B. Hofmann, Dr.P.H., FACHE, and
William A. Nelson, Ph.D.

*The viewpoints expressed by Dr. Nelson in this book do not represent those of the Veterans Health Administration.

PART I

Leadership

Understanding Your Ethical Responsibilities

Frankie Perry, FACHE

TODAY'S HEALTHCARE SYSTEM is a very complex one that's driven by many forces and weighted down by an infinite number of ethical implications. That means more ethical responsibilities for healthcare executives—responsibilities that require healthcare executives to maintain high corporate and personal ethics. These responsibilities also challenge them to balance legal and ethical parameters, act in the best interests of patients, and uphold the organization's mission, often in the face of limited resources.

How do you deal with an HIV-positive physician working with patients in your organization? What about drug and alcohol testing for your employees? Are you making the right moves to stop improper conduct, mishandling of funds, record tampering, sexual harassment, conflicts of interest? Are you meeting the healthcare needs of your community?

First, healthcare executives need to adopt an attitude that makes ethics part of their ongoing decision making and works to build a stronger, more ethically responsive healthcare system. Next, healthcare executives must take a hard look at the way they live and the way they conduct business. Part of that regimen must include an established, practical guide such as ACHE's *Code of Ethics* [see Appendix A], which embraces a professional lifestyle that embodies service, integrity, and leadership.

According to the code, healthcare executives have ethical obligations not only to the healthcare profession, but to society and community as well. These obligations also extend to the organization, the employees, the patients, and those served. It recognizes healthcare executives as the "moral agents" and business conscience of healthcare and requires them to be committed to creating "a more equitable, accessible, effective, and efficient healthcare system." When you join ACHE, you agree to abide by its *Code of Ethics*. It's your responsibility to understand this code, honor it, and to report or correct any violations. Actions of affiliates named in violation of the code are evaluated by a grievance procedure enforced by ACHE's Committee on Ethics. This includes reviewing and investigating cases and then recommending actions to the Board of Governors on allegations brought forth regarding code violations.

ACHE's Committee on Ethics annually reviews the ACHE's code to make any necessary recommendations regarding updates. In addition, the committee annually issues ethical policy statements to outline current issues and establish recommendations that healthcare executives can use.

The *Code of Ethics* and grievance procedures are included in ACHE's *Annual Report and Reference Guide*. If you have not read the code lately, please take a few minutes to do so. In addition, seek out and discuss current articles, books, conferences, and seminars about ethics with your colleagues and management team.

The place to start [strengthening and building awareness about managerial ethics] is at the ethical backbone of the healthcare management profession—ACHE's *Code of Ethics*. Remember, you represent ACHE's code. You are the example that everyone in your organization should emulate.

In Search of Internal Morality

David C. Thomasma, Ph.D.

AS INCREASING PRESSURES to compete are placed on individuals who enter the healthcare field, more and more emphasis is placed on institutional loyalty and on making tough, competitive decisions. Now is the time to examine our values and ask ourselves if we are preserving our loyalty to our patients and employees.

Healthcare executives face marketplace pressures that tell them to put survival and institutional loyalties first. But more organizations' codes of ethics and the internal morality of the profession still emphasize caring for the common good of patients. An organization's code should represent the standards of the practice agreed upon by the members, for the good of the members. It should be designed to prevent loyalties from going astray. In addition, these guidelines protect individuals from the pressures of their profession and from the improper actions of individuals in responsible positions or those to whom others entrust their lives or their fortunes.

Some typical ethical behaviors such as respecting the personhood of individuals by respecting their autonomy, telling the truth, and keeping promises can be detailed. These duties are willingly taken on by healthcare executives who, because of their commitment to those within the institution, must lead exemplary lives and

5

set the standards of behavior to be followed in the institution. There are additional ethical incentives such as respecting others, telling the truth, and keeping promises that one accepts when hired as a manager. But is there something more unique to the profession itself than these broad-based ethical obligations?

A more specific set of duties arises from the fact that healthcare executives must abide by those features of business ethics that require honesty as well as those that emphasize the internal morality of healthcare itself. According to this view, healthcare executives embrace the good of the patient as their primary value and instill that value in every aspect of institutional management. Taking this view of the profession, how can healthcare executives nurture themselves, develop their own ethics, and maintain their own posture within and on behalf of their institutions? Only persons of ethical maturity—the ability to weather criticism in order to do what is right—will successfully meet these demands.

Individuals considering any management position must have strong, delineated goals, clearly defined values, and the know-how to carry them out. These characteristics can create tremendous stress when values and ethical principles come into conflict. Leadership demands an ability to articulate how the values are in conflict and how the resolution properly respects a hierarchy of values. This ethical maturity requires that healthcare executives be selected for their commitment to the code of ethics already established for the profession. While in training, healthcare executives should study ethical quandaries faced by individuals in their profession.

Kudos to those healthcare executives who assemble with others to discuss ethical problems in management. And kudos to ACHE for inaugurating an annual ethics conference that focuses on the managerial aspects of ethical decision making in healthcare today. These are the stepping-stones we need to strengthen healthcare's internal morality.

Can a Manager Be a Moral Leader?*

John R. Griffith, FACHE

MANAGERS HAVE TWO tools for promoting moral virtue in their organizations: by example and by using the pragmatic systems of the modern organization to promote moral ends. These mechanisms are not perfect. As to whether they are effective enough to be worth the effort, the answer is that we cannot afford to find out. To be a moral leader, you have to accept the challenge.

PROMOTING VIRTUE BY EXAMPLE

Virtuous managers make moral decisions and show others that it can be done. The more positive examples there are—and the fewer negative ones—the stronger the moral culture of the organization. Recognizing virtuous decisions multiplies the effect of example by the leader. Conversely, a lack of leadership examples and of reward for virtuous decisions destroys a moral culture.

---

*This article is excerpted from *The Moral Challenges of Health Care Management* by John R. Griffith (Health Administration Press 1993).

Beyond example, the manager's pragmatic goodness allows the organization to accumulate the resources it needs to make, implement, and reward virtuous decisions. A virtuous organization is almost certainly well-run.

1. *Moral leadership is essential,* and the higher the rank of the leader the more important the moral character.
2. *Sound systems and procedures encourage virtuous acts.* Complete and accurate records, internal controls on resources, easy methods to report problems and wrongdoing, rehab programs for substance abuse, and deliberate procedures to protect individual rights all help promote moral virtue.
3. *Behavior that is not virtuous must be identified and discouraged.* The organization must express this position consistently in its policies, training programs, and operational decisions.
4. *Workers should be empowered to the greatest extent possible,* and the management style should be participative. Management should establish an environment where difficult issues can be candidly discussed.
5. *The organization should offer moral counsel and support,* beginning with first-line supervisors. Ethics committees and other resources must be available to support the supervisor and worker.
6. *The organization's visible incentives—nonmonetary and monetary—should be based on reward more than blame.* Cash rewards and prizes to the worthy may not be necessary if it is clear that they do not accrue to the unworthy.
7. *Standard methods of persuasion should be used for moral issues* as they are for other human resources concerns. An organization that deliberately promotes morality is likely to get more of it.

8. *Leadership should be selected and promoted for moral and nonmoral competence.* An organization promoting moral virtue pays competitive wages and builds an attractive work environment so it can be selective in recruitment and retention.

Obviously, this is not an easy agenda. Yet any community deserves morally excellent healthcare, and any healthcare organization can be morally improved. Building the momentum meets the moral challenge of healthcare management at its highest level.

Moral Integrity and Healthcare Leadership

David C. Thomasma, Ph.D.

THE WAY WE deliver healthcare through institutions is dramatically changing. Perhaps we are moving toward a time when healthcare will be even more highly regulated and governed than it is today.

Hospitals and home care institutions are becoming more aware that public and private expectations about the range of care to be given for specific health problems provide ambiguous support for institutional missions and philosophies. Some of these expectations are embedded in the medico-legal fabric. Others are part of the current standards of care as articulated by caregivers. For example, providing fluids and nutrition so that "nobody dies of starvation under my care" may be a common sentiment among caregivers, but it may not be legally required or morally necessary.

Since every appeal of ethical resolution cannot be tried and tested against permanently established objective rules, interpreting values, interests, and experiences are essential to the craft of management. In other words, healthcare leadership requires moral integrity. But what do we really mean when we assert that healthcare leaders must be persons of integrity? Integrity involves wholeness, predictability, and risk-taking. Wholeness is implied in the name "integrity" itself. It means that a person integrates experience, virtues, and moral rules throughout his or her career. Predictability stems from that process of integration. No one integrates experience and rules, and practice and theory, without an extensive and ongoing struggle. When we admire a person of integrity, we admire not only his or her accomplishments and levelheadedness, but also the wisdom he or she has gained from the struggle to integrate theory and practice. This struggle tests the measure of the person.

During the testing of experience and rules that occur throughout one's life, a set of fundamental, or primary, values begins to emerge from which stems predictability. These values are so profoundly a part of the person that only severe pressure can change them. For this reason, the individual who has done the hard work of establishing positions on issues is not swayed by the newest fad, the shifting sands of social mores, or the variable behavior of institutions in competitive environments.

Despite the fundamental predictability of a person who has integrity, he or she does not necessarily remain predictable in every instance. An integrated person is willing to take risks on behalf of what is right. This ability to modify one's positions is also a mark of leadership. Since the most disputed issues of our day offer the least chance of public consensus, providing leadership takes wisdom, maturity, and courage. The source of that courage lies in all the previous testing of values. Trust in his or her ability to make good decisions in the face of uncertainty helps the "predictable" person decide which values need to be preserved and which values can be placed at risk.

The habit of examining experience, interests, and moral rules does not come automatically. It must be taught by example and by training. Conferences and academic programs alike should continue to be included as a component in which leaders who have demonstrated integrity in the field of healthcare help others work through the lessons learned from past cases. Only in this way can the next generation of healthcare executives be ready to face the moral challenges of a regulated healthcare system.

Creating an
Organizational Conscience

Paul B. Hofmann, Dr.P.H., FACHE

ACROSS THE COUNTRY, the transformation of the healthcare delivery system is not occurring at the same pace. Eventually, however,
every healthcare executive will witness and, in many instances,
influence its impact. As this transition proceeds, economic and political pressures will create opportunities for innovative solutions
but, at the same time, will produce incentives that can lead to ethical dilemmas for healthcare executives.

Ultimately, it is the CEO's responsibility to establish the moral
tone of the organization. A variety of questions can and should be
raised to remind each executive that he or she will be held increasingly accountable for both personal and organizational performance from an ethical perspective. Such measurement may be implicit rather than explicit, and yet its importance is undeniable
when the moral character of leadership has become suspect in so
many fields.

BUILDING TRUST AND CONFIDENCE

How can healthcare executives merit the trust and confidence of
their colleagues and the general public? According to ACHE's *Code*

of Ethics, executives "must lead lives that embody an exemplary system of values and ethics." No one would argue with this mandate, but what system should be followed?

Familiarity with the classic theories of ethics and values is not required. Instead, as noted by the *Code of Ethics,* the executive is obligated to "conduct all personal and professional activities with honesty, integrity, respect, fairness and good faith." However, unassailable individual behavior is not enough. In view of management's power, authority, and visibility, senior management has the opportunity as well as the obligation to be consistent in their actions and provide vigorous moral leadership.

STAYING ON TRACK

In addition to displaying the virtues that others should emulate, there are two specific actions healthcare executives should consider.

Clarify organizational values. Encourage your board to develop and disseminate a value statement. Too frequently, nonsectarian organizations mistakenly believe this activity is best left to religiously sponsored organizations and serves no purpose for others.

Eventually, every healthcare system, hospital, long-term care facility, home care program, and managed care organization will be forced to make difficult resource allocation decisions involving legitimate alternatives with disparate consequences for their various constituents. When decisions such as these arise, a thorough assessment of organizational values undertaken in an objective fashion and committed to writing can serve as a valuable guide.

Produce and distribute an ethics manual. The ethics manual you produce should contain hypothetical cases depicting the broad spectrum of ethical dilemmas that could be encountered by board members, managers, physicians, employees, and volunteers. Vignettes illustrating potential conflicts of interest, possible violations of confidentiality, questionable discriminatory behavior, and comparable problems can provide instructive examples of how your organization's policies and values should be interpreted.

PROMOTE THE PROCESS

Creating and sustaining an organizational conscience is not easy. During a period when the spotlight is on all aspects of healthcare delivery, it is particularly important to promote the process.

As emphasized by ACHE's *Code of Ethics*, healthcare executives have a wide array of obligations to the profession, to patients or others served, to the organization, to employees, to the community, and to society. Although ACHE's *Code of Ethics* describes these obligations in helpful detail, it is up to healthcare executives to put these words into practice and set the organization's moral tone.

Balancing Professional and Personal Priorities

Paul B. Hofmann, Dr.P.H., FACHE

EVERY CONSCIENTIOUS HEALTHCARE executive must contend with high expectations—usually self-imposed—that create inevitable pressure to work both harder and smarter. Priorities are constantly being reassessed and shifted to accommodate new and seemingly more important requirements.

Of course, these demands aren't exclusively professional in nature. Personal and family needs invariably compete with job-related priorities for the healthcare executive's time and attention. Mere time often emerges as the healthcare executive's most precious and least available resource.

So what do we do? We compromise. Intuitively, relative costs and benefits are measured, and a choice is made. By rationalizing misjudgments and rarely acknowledging our fallibility, we manage to cope and hope that others understand. But healthcare executives have an ethical responsibility to their organizations, colleagues, and employees to do more than just cope. We must put personal issues into perspective and maintain balance to perform well professionally.

Ethical behavior has been described as obedience to the unenforceable. In addition to personal values, an executive's behavior is

17

driven by conscience, defined by the dictionary as "the inner sense of what is right or wrong in one's conduct or motives, impelling one toward right action." Consequently, there is no universal prescription healthcare executives can follow to prevent mistakes or ensure ethical behavior.

While no universal prescription exists, there are guideposts that healthcare executives can follow. For example, ACHE's *Code of Ethics*, with which all affiliates are expected to comply, contains standards of ethical behavior for healthcare executives in their professional relationships. As emphasized in the code's preamble, leaders should "merit the trust, confidence, and respect of healthcare professionals and the general public. To do so, healthcare executives must lead lives that embody an exemplary system of values and ethics." Healthcare executives should periodically review this document.

MAINTAINING BALANCE

When examining the balance between professional and personal priorities, these questions should be addressed:

- Am I eating properly, getting adequate rest and sufficient exercise, setting realistic expectations, and fostering supportive interpersonal relationships? Vitality, physical as well as mental, is an undeniable prerequisite and ongoing necessity to sustain an appropriate balance.
- Am I sensitive to emotional as well as physical warning signs of imbalance—not only in myself but in others? Am I willing to seek assistance? Healthcare organizations should provide access to counseling and other services to assist staff in addressing problems that adversely affect job performance.
- Do I resolve conflicts quickly? Honesty, commitment, trust, understanding, and accommodation are among

the many attributes required to achieve timely conflict resolution.

Historically, leaders have been more likely to monitor the behavior of subordinates and to intervene when necessary. Perhaps due to executives' perfectionist tendencies, frenetic schedules, and high energy, they are oblivious to the masochistic consequences of their behavior. Unless executives consciously and regularly examine the personal and organizational costs, along with the benefits, of professional achievement, a safe and satisfying balance will not be maintained.

Abuse of Power

Paul B. Hofmann, Dr.P.H., FACHE

As a hospital executive, I am dismayed when I see certain physicians and managers using their power to intimidate patients, families, and staff. What can I do to stop this unethical behavior and prevent it in the future?

UNFORTUNATELY, ABUSE OF power is at least as prevalent, if not more so, in healthcare organizations as it is in other types of organizations. Furthermore, because potential consequences are far more severe than in other settings, abuse of power in a clinical facility is particularly objectionable and unacceptable.

Patients and their families are exceptionally vulnerable in a time of crisis. They are apprehensive, sometimes frightened, and often intimidated by the organization's sheer physical size and bureaucratic complexity. Physicians, still at the top of the power structure in many hospitals, generally have a great deal of formal and informal organizational and personal leverage. Therefore, some individuals in authority (physicians as well as other clinical staff) may speak and act inappropriately, but this behavior is tolerated because patients and families often feel too overwhelmed and powerless to voice their objections.

Similar problems occur when managers who have significant authority do not use it for the good of the organization and those it serves. Employees under their supervision can be compromised by their misuse of power, adversely affecting both morale and productivity. Like patients and their families, employees may feel helpless and hesitant to object to such behavior.

Examples of abuse of power include rudeness, profane language, promise breaking, deception, dishonesty, and sexual harassment. Less obvious forms of abuse of power tend to be subtle and therefore more insidious; these include arrogance, use of overly confusing jargon, and withholding of information.

Management and medical staff sometimes rationalize this sort of unprofessional conduct because they view it as unintentional and nonmalicious. However, in addition to compromising its immediate victims, tolerating such behavior has several negative long-term consequences such as encouraging the individual to continue this conduct, silently condoning the behavior and suggesting to others that they can behave in a similar manner with impunity, demoralizing those who become aware of the organization's tolerance, and adversely affecting the image and reputation of the organization.

A variety of action steps can be taken to mitigate the abuse of power, including the following:

- Recognize the inadequacy of well-intentioned rhetoric, including organizational values statements unaccompanied by explicit programs to reinforce them.
- Develop and implement a code of conduct for management, staff, and physicians.
- Perform periodic ethics audits that include questions about abuse of power.
- Prepare a casebook with descriptions of unacceptable behavior and constructive interventions and use it in management orientation and training sessions.

- Conduct educational programs to promote candid discussion of these issues.
- Establish and encourage the use of a "hotline" to report inappropriate conduct.
- Sanction improper behavior promptly.
- Encourage the referral of physician problems to the medical staff's physician advisory committee.
- Emphasize the importance ofsensitivity to the values of patients, families, and staff in routine employee performance appraisals.

Regrettably, it is unlikely that you can totally prevent abuse of power, but constant vigilance and effective intervention can reduce its incidence. Most importantly, you cannot achieve this objective unless senior management and clinical leaders themselves demonstrate zero tolerance for insensitive and inappropriate behavior.

PART II

Community Relations

Healthcare Organizations' Civic Responsibilities

Paul B. Hofmann, Dr.P.H., FACHE

REGARDLESS OF ITS product or service, every employer is expected to meet basic civic responsibilities, including prompt payment of taxes, if not tax-exempt; support of charitable organizations; and participation by senior executives in local service clubs. However, healthcare organizations have unique civic obligations that exceed the conventional set of corporate responsibilities. It is the healthcare organization's ethical responsibility to take a leadership role in improving the health status of the community.

Understandably, during a period of growing financial pressures, assuming a greater role in the community can seem daunting. But this is a contribution that often requires no significant economic investment. Rather, leading the community in improving health status requires an organizational commitment of individual and collective energy.

ETHICAL CHALLENGES

Many hospitals today have an increasing proportion of their patients covered by managed care contracts, but few have a substantial portion of their revenue generated from capitation. Consequently, most hospitals are operating in an uncomfortable twilight zone, relying primarily on revenue produced by indemnity-insured patients and others for whom reimbursement is submitted on the basis of DRGS, negotiated per diem rates, or a percentage discount off charges.

As healthcare providers proceed through this challenging transition period, the number of both economic and ethical challenges grows dramatically. Managing limited resources under these circumstances creates an almost schizophrenic corporate culture. This conflict of interest is best represented by the CEO who said his most significant ethical problem is having a mission to improve the overall health of the community but being very happy when the hospital is 90 percent occupied.

RESOURCES TO GUIDE YOU

Fortunately, as efforts to improve community health status gain increasing attention, the number of resources offering guidance also grows.

Four publications deserve mention. The first is *The Healthy Communities Handbook* (National Civic League 1993). It describes an invaluable self-appraisal tool, called the "Civic Index," and explains why Jacksonville, Florida, has "one of the most forward-thinking and effective tools used in the United States to establish and monitor quality of life indicators reflective of community priorities and values." The second recommended resource is *A Handbook for Planning and Developing Integrated Delivery* (Catholic Health Association and Lewin-VHI 1993). This publication focuses on strategies for providing a continuum of comprehensive services and improving the health status of an enrolled population. The third resource is a study, "What Creates Health? Individuals and Communities Respond" (*The Healthcare Forum* 1994). It examines public values around quality of life and community health concerns. After describing emerging trends, the report presents guiding principles to encourage a new model of collaborative leadership. Finally, CEOS and their management teams will want to review ACHE's Public Policy Statement "Community Service Ethic."

If heathcare executives become more assertive in demonstrating imaginative and effective community leadership on the part of their organizations, they and their organizations will benefit. More important, the quality of community life will be enhanced.

Using Healthcare Data in Advertising

William P. Brandon, Ph.D., M.P.H.

DATA OUR ORGANIZATION has collected over the past few years indicate that we have a lower mortality rate than many of our competitor organizations. My marketing team would like to use that information—and other comparative clinical data we have collected—in an advertising campaign. What are the ethical implications of using this data for marketing purposes?

Not long ago, most healthcare advertising was considered unethical if aimed at the general public. The issues involved in the unique trust-based relationship between patients and physicians seemed to justify professional associations protecting the public with private regulation that governed professional activities and prohibited almost all advertising.

However, in recent years, the floodgates to healthcare advertising have opened. Absent intervention by organized medicine or government, advertising is the principal mechanism for addressing the unequal distribution of information between healthcare buyers and sellers. This renders genuine social benefits that may provide a moral basis for advertising.

But while many healthcare organizations are now advertising their services, few are using hard data to do so.

The tendency for healthcare organizations to use warm, fuzzy ads instead of data-based ones may partly be a remnant of the traditional prohibition against criticizing other providers. From one viewpoint, it is admirable that healthcare executives are wary of entering what is often seen as the domain of used-car salesmen and politicians.

Yet if advertising is the best way to inform consumers, and the information is accurate and relevant, why pull punches? For data to be meaningful requires valid comparisons, so it may not always be possible (or desirable) to obscure an inferior performance by competitors. For example, if one transplant facility has significantly better survival rates than another, advertising that data not only promotes the superior facility, it also provides important medical information to physicians and patients.

Many professionals fear that data about health outcomes may be misused by the media, competitors, or consumers. However, an organization can protect itself and its advertising claims by ensuring that the data meet a few basic standards.

DATA INTERPRETATIONS MUST BE HONEST

Advertising must constitute truth-telling, or it will reinforce negative stereotypes about advertising and further undermine trustworthiness in society. Therefore, advertising must not present half-truths, such as only favorable results or the positive consequences of random variation.

For example, if your organization has a lower mortality rate but the population you serve is less acutely ill than your competitor's, the mortality rate can be misleading unless it is presented in a way that acknowledges the difference in the populations.

Advertising should be based on studies by reputable third parties. For example, the Department of Health and Human Services or the National Committee for Quality Assurance (which collects HEDIS data) will produce better multi-institutional data, because they can insist on uniform definitions and procedures. Information from such sources will also be more persuasive than seemingly self-serving in-house research.

DATA MUST ADDRESS 'THE BIG PICTURE'

Finally, patient confidentiality requires that individuals must not be identifiable; however, this issue is unlikely to arise in ads involving aggregate quantitative data.

The era when physicians' superior information made them the effective decision makers has been replaced by a market regime. Now consumers must have more and better information, and advertising can help provide it. Of course, the twenty-first century may see a return to collective responsibility for the healthcare system, but in the meantime, the norms of today's healthcare marketplace justify the use of data-based advertising that accords with the guidelines above.

Publicizing Superior Care

William P. Brandon, Ph.D., M.P.H.

The cardiac center in my managed care organization has gained a stellar reputation in treating certain complex conditions, resulting in a dramatic increase in patients requiring treatment for those conditions. However, these treatments are very costly. Publicizing the availability of this excellent care is certainly in the best interest of patients, but we are concerned about cost control, as we do not wish to increase premiums. How can we strike an ethical balance?

THIS QUESTION TURNS the usual accusation against HMOs—that they succeed by enrolling the healthy and neglecting the needs of the chronically ill—on its head. Instead, it stipulates that the plan fully meets its responsibilities to those in greatest need of healthcare and then inquires about the financial implications.

The problem is that if a plan offers services for the chronically ill that are readily available and superior in quality, disproportionate numbers of sick patients are likely to join and use more health services than average patients consume. Costs will increase, leading to higher premiums. As premiums increase, relatively healthy enrollees will begin to choose competing plans whose premiums correspond more closely to the cost of the healthcare that they expect to use. This sequence of events can lead to the dreaded insurance

35

"death spiral," in which increasing premiums drive out healthy insured patients and attract only the highest-risk patients.

In reality, a single costly service is unlikely to have a significant impact on a large well-managed plan. Yet if a plan becomes recognized as providing the best care for the chronically ill across the board and entry to the plan is available after the onset of illness (e.g., in open enrollment periods with no waiting periods), adverse selection may occur.

In the scenario outlined above, the manager thinks the organization might avoid adverse selection by suppressing information about the genuine superiority of the services offered by the plan's cardiac center. Is this ethical? False or intentionally misleading information in advertisements is clearly immoral and unacceptable. In addition, healthcare regulators require that correct information flow to consumers.

But advertising aimed at securing new members need not emphasize or even mention treatments for specific health conditions. Instead, many respected plans issue ads that simply address their overall commitment to quality rather than address specific outcomes. Moreover, federal regulations require that such claims have a factual basis. Thus, while information about the plan's superior cardiac services does not have to be the focus of an advertising campaign, it can play an important role in backing up general assertions when consumers or regulators ask for specifics.

To counter the possible impact of adverse selection, the HMO manager might also promote the organization's primary care services to young families. This approach aims to neutralize any adverse selection by attracting more healthy enrollees. The organization might also contract with other health plans to provide cardiac services to their patients. Disease management is an effective way to provide high-quality, integrated, condition-specific health services to patients in a manner that yields the advantages of "outsourcing."

While healthcare organizations certainly have an ethical obligation to provide high-quality care, they are not necessarily obligated to advertise specific services. Publicizing a systemwide commitment to quality and developing strategies to avoid or offset the impact of adverse selection can allow an organization's "centers of excellence" to continue to provide superior care while keeping costs and premiums under control.

PART III

Managed Care

Ethical Issues in Managed Care

Paul B. Hofmann, Dr.P.H., FACHE

MANAGED CARE'S ECONOMIC incentives encourage health maintenance and discourage improper provision of expensive medical care. When the potential downside of managed care is acknowledged, several principal concerns usually emerge.

Historically, the most common criticism of fee-for-service payment has been an inherent financial inducement to provide more services to generate additional revenue. Physicians, of course, were not the only ones reprimanded for providing unnecessary services; hospitals and other providers receiving charge-based reimbursement were also admonished for such behavior. When the economic incentives are reversed under managed care and capitated payment, eliminating unnecessary services becomes a high priority. However, the potential for providing insufficient care cannot be ignored. Therefore, the first and most prominent concern about managed care is the specter of undertreatment.

A second major ethical problem is the exclusion of high-risk patients. Currently, enrollment in managed care plans is mainly limited to employed individuals who are at least healthy enough to work. Therefore, people with debilitating chronic conditions are essentially excluded from these plans. This problem will be largely addressed if universal access is guaranteed as part of healthcare reform.

A third concern is the issue of confidentiality. As managed care programs and their databases expand, the volume of information maintained on individual subscribers will become increasingly detailed and more in demand. Consequently, preserving an individual's right to privacy will become a difficult ethical challenge.

Another problem involves the increasing reliance on practice guidelines and protocols to determine approval or rejection of treatment requests by managed care representatives. Such tools are reasonable as long as they contribute to promoting efficient coordination of cost-effective services. Misuse of protocols occurs when there is 1) an extended delay in obtaining a decision; 2) inordinate medical influence being exercised by nonphysicians; 3) insensitivity to individual circumstances, which results in general conformity at the price of mediocrity; and 4) denial of legitimate therapeutic services to patients. At substantial ethical risk are professional and personal values as well as patient welfare.

Thus, to further ensure that managed care works in the best interest of all those concerned, healthcare executives should: reinforce existing quality assurance programs; establish procedures to monitor and evaluate denials of treatment coverage; strengthen policies to avoid unauthorized access to confidential patient information; and encourage the cautious development, refinement, and acceptance of practice guidelines.

Managed care raises other ethical questions for executives in hospitals and health networks. For example, is the organization accepting significant responsibility for meeting community healthcare needs? Is improved health status the ultimate goal? Explicit values must be reflected in system design considerations so that the consumer's role in decision making, within the constraints of a managed care environment, is not compromised. Similarly, given the aggressive pursuit of many organizations to build physician alliances, healthcare executives must be certain that their criteria for success include specific measures of public as well as organizational benefit.

Caught Between
Two Paradigms

Paul B. Hofmann, Dr.P.H., FACHE

THE MOVEMENT TOWARD managed care in the United States is clearly accelerating, and almost every institutional and individual provider has some proportion of patients who are members of a health plan paying substantially less than full charges for the care received.

Differences also appear to exist in treatment patterns for managed care enrollees as compared with patients covered by indemnity insurance. Both proponents and opponents of managed care point to studies showing that managed care patients not only have fewer admissions and shorter lengths of stay than traditional insurance patients, but when admitted, account for lower charges and receive fewer intensive care services. One such study, conducted at BayState Medical Center, Springfield, Massachusetts, and based on a cross-sectional analysis of consecutive intensive care unit admissions (controlled for case mix and severity of illness), found that for medical and emergency surgical patients, managed care patients spent about 35 percent less time in the ICU. And yet, importantly, there was no apparent difference in mortality or ICU readmission.

While managed care's critics contend that it provides incentives for substandard care, studies such as the one noted above suggest that quality of care need not be adversely affected. Ensuring that quality of care is not affected by managed care is the ethical imperative of both the organizational and individual provider. Regardless of the way care is managed, all patients should receive one standard of care.

In quite basic terms, the organization's responsibility is to ensure that sufficient resources are available to facilitate optimal care and that economic incentives do not supplant the organization's mission of improving community health status. In turn, individual providers must be vigilant about putting their patients' medical needs above all else. While few would argue with these imperatives, upholding them is admittedly no small feat. Those who have succeeded attribute their success to their commitment to the patient and to reexamining and making fundamental changes to those aspects of their activity that do not adversely affect patient care.

Those who operate in a primarily fee-for-service environment must guard against the provision of inefficient, unnecessary, overpriced, and inappropriate medical services. These are certainly the most common criticisms of such a system. In turn, if you or your organization provide managed care, you must be vigilant about ensuring that your plan does not:

- cause anxiety and inconvenience patients;
- create an excessive administrative burden for practitioners and institutional providers;
- deny reimbursement for potentially life-saving treatment
- exclude competent providers;
- provide incentives for withholding care; and
- unnecessarily restrict patient choice of providers.

At the same time, you must make an investment in your managed care program, particularly in the primary care physicians who serve as gatekeepers. If they are expected to decrease referrals to specialists, you have an ethical responsibility to ensure that they have the appropriate level of training to care for a broader spectrum of patient ills. Further, it is critical that they share your commitment to the patient and are comfortable assuming frontline responsibility for the equitable distribution of resources.

Given the above challenges, the degree of organizational and personal angst in healthcare is understandably high. Our job is to make sure that these fears are unfounded and that neither patients nor providers are compromised.

The Ethics of Managed Care

Jane Fulton, Ph.D.

I am a senior manager in a managed care organization. Patients and physicians often tell me they think that managed care is unethical because it denies necessary treatment. How can I respond to these charges? What can my organization do to ensure that physicians and staff continue to provide appropriate care and service in this managed care environment?

WHEN WE CHANGE the rules of a system that has been in place for many years, there is bound to be some controversy. Controversy, and the complaints and concerns generated by such changes, are often tied to our concepts of fairness and duty—concepts that are fundamental to ethics. Understanding the ethics of managed care requires us to understand the individual ethics and perspectives of the parties involved.

THE PHYSICIAN ETHIC

Most physicians practicing today were trained to be patient advocates. They have been taught that a physician's duty is to rally resources for the patient's benefit, and in the past, health insurance provided the financial back-up for this care. Today, that duty still is

49

the concept that underlies the physician ethic of patient care. However, many physicians feel that the principles of managed care make it difficult for them to fulfill their advocacy role.

THE MANAGEMENT ETHIC

For healthcare executives, times have also changed. Gone are the days when our job of resource allocation had no real limit. The management ethic today is founded in distributive justice, where healthcare executives try to allocate limited resources as fairly as possible. Managers must juggle highly sensitive cost-benefit issues daily.

ADDRESSING THESE CONCERNS

Based on their education, training, and fundamental beliefs, most physicians and managers want to—and do—behave ethically. Therefore, the challenge in managed care organizations is not necessarily to ensure that their physicians and managers continue to do so, but rather to provide them with the assurance that the treatments, protocols, and duties they must carry out under a managed care system are fair and ethical.

To do this, an organization must achieve an "ethical consensus," so that the managers' need to align cost and appropriate care aligns with the physicians' need to honor their duty to provide care and advocacy for the patient. One way to accomplish this is to actively involve physicians and other key providers in the development and implementation of accepted care paths and protocols. If healthcare executives and physicians are able to collaborate to develop, agree upon, and formally approve the components of the care paths and protocols, healthcare executives can determine cost-benefit issues involved in each component early in the process. Also, physicians will be able to use treatment protocols that they themselves have approved and will be able to use the research evidence for each standard to describe probabilities of risk and expected outcomes to patients.

SUSTAINING ETHICS

Managed care has gained a reputation for being "cheap"—for trying to spend less at the expense of patient care quality. Rather than continuing the historical pattern of spending more, those of us in healthcare management need to build a plan to spend smarter and reinforce the benefits of such a plan with staff. This will be the only way our field can sustain a trend of cost control and still be recognized as ethical.

PART IV

Mergers and Integration

Pick Your Partners Wisely

Paul B. Hofmann, Dr.P.H., FACHE

A 1995 *NEW YORK TIMES* article highlighted the turn of events surrounding the merger between a small, nonsectarian community hospital and a nearby larger Roman Catholic hospital. The merger has since resulted in a lawsuit by several family planning groups, who contend that the merger limits patients' access to contraception, abortion referrals, and related counseling services.

Although the lawsuit is apparently the first of its kind in the country, it is an important reminder of the potential impact of merger, affiliation, and frankly any partnership arrangements that our organizations are considering. Decisions made in the interest of continued organizational viability are also likely to have a profound impact on the communities we serve.

Only in extreme cases will failure to consider the impact of our partnership decisions on the community result in legal action, but they will most certainly result in a crisis of confidence. For that reason, when choosing your partners, you will want to consider the following questions:

Although subjective when compared to a review of balance sheets, examining the relative compatibility of each organization's vision, mission, and values is imperative. A failure to explore real or potential conflicts in this area can severely compromise the effective integration of two distinct corporate cultures. The example above illustrates the issues that can arise when a Catholic hospital and nonsectarian hospital merge. But what about the merger between an investor-owned organization and a not-for-profit? How will their respective missions and values be affected? What compromises and concessions can and should these organizations make? Both parties must revisit what they hope to accomplish through merger, acquisition, or affiliation and weigh the benefits and chances for success against the opportunity costs involved.

WHAT ARE THE IMPLICATIONS OF THE PROPOSED
PARTNERSHIP FOR THE COMMUNITY?

Beyond determining the economic implications of your partnership, measure the impact it will have on the community. What effect will duplication or consolidation of services have? Can the new medical staff meet community needs? Is it possible or reasonable to preserve the heritage or identity of each organization?

To determine community need and to achieve buy-in of all stakeholders, a meeting of legitimate stakeholders should be held to share what you hope to accomplish. Participants should include board members, senior executives, physicians, and employees. It may also be beneficial to invite major donors, employers, health plan representatives, and community leaders to obtain their support as well as learn of any reservations they may have about the proposed partnership.

Assuming you have the support of stakeholders, developing a comprehensive action plan to address their pivotal concerns throughout the merger, acquisition, or affiliation process can dramatically reduce disillusionment and help maintain commitment. Most important, this action plan should promote realistic expectations of the new organization.

Taking the above issues into consideration will improve the degree of cooperation and compromise essential to accomplishing your ultimate objectives. Evaluating organizational fit and assessing, generating, and maintaining commitment to the partnership may prove as vital to the partnership's long-term success as obtaining compliance with legal and other requirements.

Handling Job Uncertainty During a Merger

Marc D. Hiller, Dr.P.H.

I am the CEO of a hospital that is considering a merger with another healthcare organization. At this point, it is unclear which CEO will retain the position should the merger take place. How do I balance my personal concerns about career stability with my responsibility to my organization?

IF I PUT myself in this CEO's shoes, at a glance the answer seems simple: My first and foremost ethical responsibility is to my organization and those whom it serves-the community, patients, and employees. Yet, given a second look, this situation presents anything but a simple problem.

While I seek to advance my hospital's mission in accordance with my ethical obligations as described in ACHE's *Code of Ethics,* I cannot ignore the reality of the potential impact of the pending merger on my personal life. A host of potentially competing personal concerns may demand my attention:

- What should I expect from the new organization?
- If I do not emerge as the CEO, how will my self-image, not to mention my professional reputation, be affected?

- What would the loss of this position mean to my family and our financial security?
- Must I choose between what I know is "right" for my organization and what I feel personally, in terms of self-interest, my ego, and my drive to be named the new CEO?

The dilemma may be further exacerbated if the mission of the new organization is grounded on markedly different values (e.g., teaching vs. charity mission, investor-owned vs. community not-for-profit, religious vs. nonsectarian). What if this new mission, while both organizationally and ethically sound, is in conflict with my personal value set? To CEOs making such a decision, I recommend:

Be honest and sincere. Recognize any uncertainty and acknowledge your personal needs and the needs of your family. Do not deceive yourself or others. Convey your concerns and expectations to your board.

Maintain self-confidence. Recognize that your knowledge, experience, unique expertise, and skills go with you wherever you may go. Your professional stature and reputation should, if the need arises, help you secure a healthcare executive position with another organization.

Be a good steward. Maintain an unselfish commitment to the welfare of others and the new organization's success. Recognize that your primary obligation, whether in your former organization or the emerging one, is to manage the organization in a prudent and responsible manner regarding the rights of society, the community, those who developed the organization, and those who will inherit it in the future.

Expect what is fair from your board. To ensure your actions are not unduly clouded by your personal concerns for job security, negotiate a just compensation package or separation agreement on the chance that you do not remain in the new organization.

Maintain loyalty and integrity. Your underlying moral principles should be compatible with those of the new organization. You should be able to be faithful and devoted to its values, ethics, founding principles, mission, and priorities. If that is not the case, however, you should take yourself out of the running for CEO.

In closing, remember that with most ethical dilemmas there is no right or wrong solution, and there is seldom a solution that will please everyone: your organization, your family, and you. In working through difficult situations, the goal is to carefully examine all of the angles and determine which solution is most compatible with your organizational responsibilities and your personal convictions.

Executive Incentives in Organizational Mergers and Acquisitions

Paul B. Hofmann, Dr.P.H., FACHE

MY ORGANIZATION WILL probably be acquired by another organization, and I have been offered an incentive by that organization to support the transaction. I believe the outcome will benefit both entities, but am I ethically obligated to disclose the incentive?

Although there has been a slight decline in the number of healthcare mergers and acquisitions, consolidation within the field is far from over. Because clear support from senior management can be a decisive factor in the success of a consolidation, it is not surprising that incentives are sometimes offered. These incentives could take several forms, including a specific dollar payment; appointment as the CEO or COO of the new entity; an executive position elsewhere within the system, an attractive consulting arrangement; or a generous severance/retirement package (i.e., a "golden parachute").

Ethically, you are plainly obligated to disclose to the board the incentive that you were offered. By revealing a potential conflict of interest, you have acknowledged that your support for the merger may be influenced by the incentive. Indeed, the proposed transaction may unequivocally benefit your current organization as well, but inevitably, you must decide where your loyalties lie.

It is simplistic to suggest that your loyalty should be to your organization. After all, your organization consists of your board, medical staff, employees, and, if investor-owned, your shareholders. The needs and interests of these various constituents are probably different, rather than totally aligned. Further, you must consider your obligation to other stakeholders—your family, your administrative staff, patients, the community, and previous donors to the organization. You could, of course, refuse to accept the incentive, making a concerted effort to remain completely impartial and objective. While this decision may be in your organization's best interest, it might not be in your personal interest. So, what should you do?

Regardless of whether you accept or reject the incentive, you should disclose it to your board. Ideally, you and your board have established and maintained a solid relationship based upon mutual trust and confidence. The absence or deterioration of either of these during merger negotiations can jeopardize a transaction as quickly as unanticipated legal or financial obstacles can. Although you could conceal the incentive and hope that it does not become known and adversely affect existing or proposed relationships, this is a risky and possibly illegal strategy.

It is generally preferable to address potential problems before they arise. In this situation, two options are available, and they are not mutually exclusive. The first is to negotiate an acquisition protection clause in your employment contract. For example, the language might specify that a severance package would be activated if you were not appointed to CEO or to another acceptable position in the merged entity that included your organization. Pension and other benefits should also be covered. The board should be cautious not to make the acquisition protection clause too beneficial, and thus inadvertently provide an incentive for you to leave the organization. A second option is to suggest that a separate agreement be negotiated to encourage you to remain with the organization during the transition, regardless of your eventual position—if any—within the new entity. This retention bonus should motivate you to continue promoting the organization's best interest and discourage your premature departure.

While the above two approaches are options, the following action is not. Your organization must have a comprehensive board policy that recognizes that the CEO is not the only likely recipient of an incentive proposal. In the past, board members, their immediate families, and other senior executives have been offered inducements to support hospital mergers and acquisitions. Conflict disclosure policies and procedures have become mandated to minimize and, preferably, prevent improper conduct in a variety of areas.

Financial or other incentives to influence decisions and behavior are not inherently inappropriate. The Internal Revenue Service has provided clear guidelines for a "conflicts of interest" policy. According to the IRS, the policy should require disclosure by interested parties of financial interests and all related material facts. It should also contain procedures for:

- determining whether the financial interest of the concerned party may result in a conflict of interest;
- addressing an identified conflict of interest; and
- applying the policy to a compensation committee.

In addition to stipulating adequate record keeping, the policy should ensure distribution to all trustees, officers, and members of committees with board-delegated powers. Lastly, there is a requirement to obtain an annual conflict-of-interest statement from these individuals. The creation of this conflict-of-interest policy should:

- stimulate thoughtful deliberation about various scenarios;
- identify possible inducements and recipients;

- remind key stakeholders of their ethical and legal obligations;
- encourage individuals to fulfill their fiduciary responsibilities; and
- promote behavior consistent with the mission, vision, and values of the organization.

The purpose of this process is to help eliminate ambiguities and the rationalizations that otherwise conscientious leaders might use to defend their actions. The fundamental ethical imperative will always be prompt and full disclosure.

PART V

Use of Information

Respecting Proprietary Information (A)

Gary Edwards, J.D.

I recently went to work for a competitor of my former employer and have been asked to play a major role in crafting my new organization's strategic plan. Since I was also intimately involved in developing my former employer's strategic plan, I question how much of that information is proprietary and how much is acceptable to share with my new colleagues.

MOST HEALTHCARE ORGANIZATIONS consider a variety of business information to be proprietary and confidential, including cost and pricing data, patient records, customer and supplier lists, and the organization's strategic plans. Similarly, your former employer quite likely regards its current and past strategic plans as proprietary as well.

When you joined that organization, or perhaps later when you were first given access to proprietary or confidential information, you may have signed a confidentiality or nondisclosure agreement that formally prohibited you from sharing such information with anyone outside the organization. Even if your employer failed to execute such an agreement, you have an ethical responsibility not to disclose information that the organization considered to be proprietary and treated in such a manner.

69

It is also possible that your previous employer's strategic business plan, or important information about it, may have lost its proprietary status if, for instance, the plan has been shared with key suppliers, competitors, or other businesses with whom your previous employer was partnering or contracting without obtaining nondisclosure agreements. If the organization has not been careful to protect its proprietary information, under some circumstances its negligence may cause the information to lose its proprietary character. Regardless, you should not take the liberty of disclosing such information.

Assuming that the strategic plan has been properly handled and protected, however, it may contain important information that is not confidential. For instance, strategic planning typically includes analyses of competitors based on publicly available information and market research. Although you are not entitled to take information directly from your former employer, you can exercise the skills that you developed there to efficiently gather and analyze similar information for your current employer, including information about your former organization.

Similarly, the strategic plan will be predicated on an understanding of past, present, and prospective customers, their needs, priorities, and resources. Here, the greater challenge may be distinguishing between what you know by virtue of having been in the field for some years and what you know that your former employer would consider proprietary information.

If you are uncertain about this or other information that might be proprietary, ask yourself the following questions:

- Could my former employer reasonably consider this information to be proprietary in nature?
- If I were in my former employer's place, would I consider this information to be proprietary?

If your answer to either of these questions is "yes," do not disclose the information. If you feel uncertain about the status of information, seek competent legal counsel.

Over the years, I have participated in discussions of strategic planning and competitive intelligence with more than 100 corporate clients. My experience has taught me two things relevant to this question. First, most executives would be delighted to know the details of the strategic plans of their major competitors. Second, nearly all of those executives have told me that knowing the specifics of their competitors' plans would unlikely affect their own. Organizational success depends on understanding your market, being close to your customers, and maintaining a reputation for quality and integrity. You do need to understand the competition and its strategy, but you will find that understanding in the market, not in your competitor's proprietary information.

Respecting Proprietary Information (B)

Joan Elise Dubinsky, Esq.

I am a senior manager, recently laid off due to a restructuring. One of my former organization's major competitors has offered me a position. I was not required to sign a noncompete agreement with my former employer, but I am wondering what my ethical obligations are regarding use of proprietary information in my new position.

THIS SITUATION REPRESENTS a common ethical dilemma—the difference between what you have the right to do and the right thing to do. However, the answer to this one is relatively easy: In short, the ethical manager respects proprietary information regardless of a legally binding noncompete agreement.

Let's face it—no one enjoys layoffs. Organizations implement layoffs only as last-ditch efforts when faced with severe economic pressures. No practical healthcare organization incorporates layoffs into its normal workforce strategy. It hurts to lay off staff and it hurts to be laid off.

The emotional and ethical challenges facing laid-off executives are well known. Laid-off managers may doubt their value as professionals and question whether they can support their families. They face another classic ethical dilemma when job hunting: Do I tell the truth about being laid off or do I "sugar-coat" the situation to avoid prejudicing my next employer? Even in the most civil and well-managed layoff situation, the departing manager may be angry.

This very anger can lead some executives to consider less-than-ethical behavior. It can be tempting to take proprietary information with you on the last day of your old job. Patient lists, physician practice agreements, pricing schedules, audit reports, business plans, and marketing strategies are examples of proprietary information that is valuable to both the old and the new employer. Indeed, some departing employees believe that they will be more attractive to their next employer if they take some of this information as they go.

Proprietary information is a type of property, valuable precisely because it is secret. It takes labor to create property, and therefore the creators of that property have the right to what they have made. We generally accept that the one who does the work (or creates the information) should reap the benefit.

In the highly competitive world of healthcare, one HMO's confidential marketing strategies could be very valuable to similar organizations wishing to expand into the same areas. The creator of the proprietary information has a right to keep it secret and protect it from use by others.

Savvy organizations ask for non-compete agreements from key staff in an effort to keep certain information secret. The typical non-compete agreement protects more than healthcare "secrets," however. The standard clause reads: "For six months after I leave my employment here, I will not work in St. Louis for a healthcare organization that directly competes with my employer." These agreements tend to restrict an executives' choices in *where* they will work next, *when* they will work there, and *what* they may do.

The goals of most noncompete agreements are threefold:

1. To protect investment in key staff by making job-hopping unattractive

2. To limit costs for recruitment and training
3. To keep certain information secret by limiting the opportunities where an executive would be tempted to reveal proprietary information

The ethical obligations with regard to enforceable non-compete agreements are straightforward. Ethical managers keep the promises they have made. They may not reveal confidential, proprietary, and trade secret information. They can take with them and freely use at their next jobs any general knowledge or skills acquired while working for their former employer. They may not use the former employer's proprietary information for any purpose—unless the former employer grants permission.

Without an enforceable agreement, is there still an underlying obligation to respect the "secrets" of a former employer? Most business ethicists, and even some judges, would answer that question with a resounding "yes." The obligation to protect proprietary information arises from the nature of the information itself, not the existence of an agreement.

When leaving one job and taking the next, a responsible health-care executive continues to protect the proprietary information of his or her former employer. This obligation runs in parallel to the duty to protect the proprietary information of the new employer. Though it may seem slightly contradictory, executives must learn to safeguard the proprietary "secrets" of many organizations often simultaneously.

To paraphrase Mark Twain, who opined that Wagner's music was better than it sounds, this issue is really more straightforward than it seems.

PART VI

Human Resources

Ethical Duties to Employees

David C. Thomasma, Ph.D.

A DRAMATIC SHIFT has occurred. What was once a one-on-one doctor-patient relationship now includes a myriad of third parties— not only the payers but also staff, nurses, specialists, quality control experts, and many others. Ensuring the quality and ethics of care practiced in institutions is now the responsibility of many persons [see Appendix B3].

Today, institutions are held publicly accountable in moral and legal terms for the quality and effectiveness of the care provided. Such a radical transformation can lead to a sense of loss of control over the standards of care, since so many individuals are now responsible for the outcome. Hence, a paradigm shift has occurred. The individual doctor-patient relationship must be rethought to delivery of care as a community of caregivers, with third-party interests, working within a close-knit and mutually supportive environment. When any part of this dynamic fails, the quality of care and the moral stature of the institution collapses. Ultimately the buck must stop with the healthcare executive.

Most executives are reluctant to address a problem until it occurs, understandably preferring to work on the myriad of current problems and challenges that beset every institution. This tendency is analogous to that of modern medicine, which prefers intervention to prevention. In the end, more damage is done by not anticipating and addressing potential problems. Ethical standards of practice do not just happen automatically. They require explicit attention, articulation, education, practice, reinforcement, and rewards.

The healthcare organization itself must be managed with consistently high ethical and professional standards. The healthcare executive, acting with other appropriate responsible parties, must ensure an environment conducive for carrying out the task of quality healthcare and for accomplishing the mission, philosophy, and goals of the individual institution. All healthcare executives have an ethical and professional obligation to employees. Some of these obligations encompass:

- Creating a working environment conducive to underscoring employee ethical conduct and behavior
- Ensuring that individuals may freely express their ethical concerns without prejudice to their jobs
- Providing mechanisms for discussion of such concerns, and for addressing and redressing them, so that employees know where to turn for support
- Establishing procedures for the resolution of ethical dilemmas through consensus building or other methodologies
- Committing the institution to ethical standards in the community, even in the midst of competition that might threaten to erode some of those standards in the interests of expediency
- Working with other healthcare institutions to help formulate a national policy about healthcare access, so that the survival of the institution is not at stake when care is given to the poor and needy

In these ways, commitments are made to the employees, staff, and management of an institution, ensuring that their work and values for the good of patients and the community will not be torpedoed by unethical practices. These commitments represent the moral center of the enterprise that is healthcare delivery today.

Avoiding Sexual Harassment in the Workplace

Marc D. Hiller, Dr.P.H.

DEBATE OVER THE issue of sexual harassment has found its way onto the front pages of newspapers and into the board rooms, executive offices, cafeterias, and hallways of organizations around the country.

WHAT IS SEXUAL HARASSMENT?

Sexual harassment in the extreme form is the intimidation of subordinates by those in power or authority in order to exact sexual favors that ordinarily would not be granted.

Sexual harassment in the workplace may involve the threat to the victim's professional advancement, salary increase, or continued employment. In more subtle forms, sexual harassment can include use of profane language or inappropriate body language. While harassment of males does occur, harassment of females is more common.

From an ethical perspective, sexual harassment is morally wrong and constitutes unacceptable, unprofessional behavior. Sexual harassment is harmful to women as individuals because it blatantly violates the victim's personal autonomy and sense of equality. The victim is also degraded and may be coerced into action or unjustly denied professional advancement. Harassment is harmful to women as a whole because it further precipitates the sexual stereotypes that make it difficult, if not impossible, for women to be judged in the workplace on the basis of performance, intelligence, and skill.

ROLES AND RESPONSIBILITIES

In today's healthcare organizations, male and female employees work, travel, dine, and fraternize together. In addition, female employees typically outnumber males and are often in subordinate positions. For these reasons, the management team is more likely to face situations involving sexual harassment.

When harassment does occur, the management team is morally bound to respond quickly to convey to the organization that the behavior will not be tolerated or condoned. The hospital's management team must also know what steps to take to avoid or minimize any legal action against the organization.

Because the management team plays a leadership role in setting the values and moral climate for an organization, they are responsible for maintaining a work environment free of sexual harassment. In accepting the moral responsibility to put an end to harassment in the workplace, the management team must:

- acknowledge that sexual harassment can occur in their organizations, openly deal with it, and focus efforts on prevention;
- provide employee training programs that heighten awareness about sexual harassment;
- formulate a firm policy statement against harassment and communicate it to employees at all levels in the organization through both formal and informal channels;
- establish organizationwide, anti-harassment policies in an effort to secure compliance;

- investigate all complaints of alleged sexual harassment thoroughly and fairly, taking appropriate action against offenders;
- establish a course of action through which sexual harassment can be reported while preserving the personal dignity, self-esteem, and respect of the victim; and
- use staff exit interviews, preferably conducted by an executive of the same gender, to determine whether the staff member's dismissal or decision to resign was not predicated on advances by a superior.

These strategies will convey to organizations that immoral practices will not be sanctioned in our healthcare organizations.

Examining Hiring Practices

Paul B. Hofmann, Dr.P.H., FACHE

EXECUTIVES IN HEALTHCARE organizations as well as other fields should recognize that compliance with the many legal and regulatory requirements pertaining to hiring and terminating practices is only the beginning, not the end, of an organization's ethical obligation to deal fairly with its potential and current staff. The recruitment, screening, and selection of new personnel must be conducted in a manner that is consistent with both implicit and explicit organizational values.

RECRUITMENT

It may be tempting to depict an organization in an usually favorable light by minimizing political and other problems, particularly in recruiting for positions at a senior level. Inevitably, conveying an unrealistic profile of the existing environment and/or concealing specific problems will damage the credibility of whomever is involved; the truth will eventually become obvious to the new staff member and no one will be well served by this type of subterfuge. Lack of full disclosure is deceptive and clearly unethical.

The retention of a search firm to assist in the recruitment process does not eliminate the need for complete candor in discussing potential problems related to a position. Similarly, overly optimistic projections of opportunities for promotion, salary increases, additional space and capital, expanded staff support, or other resource commitments are seductive and indefensible. This discussion would be incomplete without reference to the topics of equal opportunity and affirmative action. Racial and gender discrimination still exists in the healthcare field, as it does in other professions, and substantive progress toward eliminating discrimination is prevented by rhetoric about advances made. Ultimately, the CEO is responsible for addressing previous inequities by creating and sustaining a corporate culture that actively recruits and develops qualified minorities and women. Formal steps should be taken to encourage these candidates, both internal and external, to apply for the position.

SCREENING AND SELECTION

Among the ethical concerns involved in the screening and selection process is determining how internal candidates will be considered. First, there should be no question regarding an internal candidate's right to apply for a different position in the organization. Although individuals currently performing at exceptional levels may be ideally suited for their current positions, it is unethical to deny them fair consideration.

The method of evaluating candidates is another critical factor with moral overtones. For example, not only should the questions asked of candidates be fair and free from gender and racial bias, but the same questions should be asked of all candidates. In addition, if group interviews are conducted, an objective rating system will ensure a nonprejudicial assessment.

An organization's awareness of its ethical obligation to its employees and potential employees is the first step in ensuring fair treatment of candidates in the recruitment, screening, and selection processes.

Impaired Healthcare Executives

Frankie Perry, FACHE

SOCIETY EXPECTS CERTAIN individuals in certain walks of life to conform to certain behaviors. Police officers are expected to abide by the law. Teachers are expected to make the pursuit of knowledge an empathic quest. Artists are expected to appreciate the aesthetic nature of things. And healthcare executives are expected to practice the standards of good health they advocate for the public.

Those running this country's healthcare institutions are not expected to poorly manage their own health. But when they fall victim to substance abuse, mental and emotional instability, or senility and continue to conduct business as usual, they do more than diminish their own public image. Impaired healthcare executives can also damage the public image of their organizations of employment.

Impairment typically leads to misconduct in the form of incompetence and unsafe or unprofessional behavior, leading to loss of productivity and errors in judgment. Such behaviors can have a substantial negative effect on an organization's bottom line. It follows that public confidence in an organization led by an impaired executive can be diminished if it appears the organization is not being managed with consistently high standards of professional and ethical practice. This lack of public confidence can profoundly affect an organization. Communities are compelled by logic, hard

89

pressed to support an organization—including healthcare organizations—that they deem unworthy of their support.

ACHE recognizes that impairment in the form of alcoholism, chemical dependency, mental and emotional instability, or senility is a problem that affects all of society—including its own ranks. ACHE knows that such problems cut across the boundaries of age and profession. But ACHE does more than acknowledge this condition; it seeks to address it [see Appendix B4]. In fact, ACHE's very own *Code of Ethics* states that "healthcare executives have an obligation to act in ways that will merit the trust, confidence, and respect of healthcare professionals and the public. To do this, healthcare executives must lead lives that embody an exemplary system of values and ethics." ACHE believes that all healthcare executives have an obligation to do the following:

- Maintain a personal health status that is free from impairment.
- Refrain from all professional activities if impaired.
- Expeditiously seek a cure if impairment occurs.
- Urge impaired colleagues to expeditiously seek a cure and to refrain from all professional activities while impaired.
- Report the impairment to the appropriate person or persons, should the colleague refuse to seek professional assistance and should the state of impairment persist.
- Recommend or provide, within one's employing organization, avenues for reporting impairment and either access or referral to treatment or assistance programs.
- Urge the community to provide information and resources for assistance and treatment of alcoholism, substance abuse, mental and emotional instability, and senility as needed and appropriate.

Through these commitments, ACHE seeks to ensure that the good of patients and the community remains the top priority of every healthcare executive.

Ensuring Fair
Termination Procedures

Paul B. Hofmann, Dr.P.H., FACHE

WHEN HEALTHCARE EXECUTIVES are faced with a termination decision, a number of issues arise. Although many of these issues are legal ones, a number of critical ethical considerations must be made as well.

The potential for violating ethical standards exists both before and after an employee's termination. Throughout the discharge process, it is the healthcare executive's responsibility to act in the organization's best interest while ensuring that the employee is treated fairly.

Because the imposition of any sanction, particularly termination, is uncomfortable for all parties, there is an undeniable tendency to procrastinate and rationalize reasons for doing so. However, neither the organization nor the individual involved is well served by a failure to confront a discharge situation in a timely manner.

The organization's effectiveness is compromised by the performance of a marginal employee. The credibility of the manager is damaged by a perceived weakness to act promptly. And the employees working with or being supervised by the individual in question are certainly affected adversely. Further, if the decision to act is made late and a wrongful termination charge is filed, ethically and legally the decision maker is vulnerable if performance discussions and related events have not been documented.

In addition to facing discharge decisions regarding poor-performing individuals, healthcare executives continue to gain painful experience in making layoff decisions. Because personnel cutbacks may become increasingly necessary, a comprehensive plan for conducting layoffs is essential.

The ethical issues involved in laying off healthcare staff are no different than those for employees in other fields. Therefore, the plan should emphasize such fundamentals as:

- provision of timely, accurate information—control rumors by keeping personnel informed;
- fulfillment of salary and benefit commitments; and
- meaningful outplacement assistance.

It is critical to remember that whether terminating an employee or planning, announcing, and implementing layoffs, the healthcare executive's actions will have profound and pervasive implications for not only these individuals but for the staff who remain. The need for ethical sensitivity in these matters cannot be overstated.

TERMINATION FOLLOW-UP

Virtually all senior executives have, at one time or another, experienced ambivalence about the type and extent of reference information to release about terminated employees. Confirming only the dates of employment may minimize time, energy, and possible liability, but, under most circumstances, taking such a stance is unreasonable and unnecessary. Honesty and relevancy are the underlying principles that should guide the release of all information. If these two criteria are met, an executive will have complied with a professional and ethical obligation to be responsive.

Obviously, when a discharge has been contentious, particular caution should be exercised in answering questions. As a general guideline, if the truth might harm the candidate's job prospects, the information can be provided if it was shared previously with the discharged employee and, preferably, documented.

Restrictions on a reference are greatest when a formal, written agreement with the discharged employee specifies what can be released. In such a situation, no discretion or judgments are entailed; the legal requirements are clear, and no ethical dilemma exists.

Accepting Vendor Gifts

Gary Edwards, J.D.

A vendor recently offered me four tickets to a Chicago Bulls game. I am the vendor's primary contact in our organization, so I was wondering if the tickets are something I should refuse, something I can use myself, or something that I should pass over to my organization?

BOTH THE GIVING and receiving of gifts, gratuities, and entertainment between parties in a business relationship pose difficult questions of policy and practice. Most organizations have written standards to guide business ethics and conduct. Nearly all of these companies address the receipt of gifts by their own employees; however, the standards vary from absolute prohibition to reciprocity to what is "reasonable" and "appropriate" in the judgment of the recipient.

Let's consider the purpose of business gifts, the possible motives of giver and recipient, and what is at stake for both parties. Many business people, especially those in sales and marketing, view gifts, gratuities, and entertainment as ways of building a relationship with a customer. Others, including professional buyers and business owners, see the practice as barely distinguishable from bribery.

If "building a relationship" with a customer means better understanding their business and its needs in order to do a superior job of anticipating and meeting those needs, then some type of gift may provide valuable opportunities for achieving that objective. For example, a business lunch following a customer site visit might allow more time for discussion and questions about the customer's operations than a brief conversation in a busy office.

It is much more difficult, however, to see how gifts and favors contribute to a relationship of trust and understanding. If a vendor provides a customer with four tickets to a Chicago Bulls game, what kind of relationship is the vendor trying to advance? This is not an opportunity for better understanding the business needs of a customer. It is much more likely an attempt to undermine the independent, objective judgment that every employee owes his or her employer, an attempt to ingratiate oneself and to create a preference, or even an effort to create a sense of obligation on the part of the customer.

What about the vendor who simply wants to say "Thanks for doing business with my organization"? Genuine gratitude and courtesy are as welcome in business as they are anywhere. Appropriateness of expression is critical, however. If gratitude is meant to be shown by a gift, then the gift should be corporate not personal. A promotional product or service or a special discount can each be valued ways of expressing gratitude to an organization. But gifts that are intended for the personal benefit of an employee can convey the impression that the vendor is seeking to buy favor and undermine judgment.

In this case, you might tell the vendor that you will pass on the gift to the organization and the tickets will be given out via an employee drawing or some other mechanism. That way, you are not only acting ethically, you are also sending a message to the vendor that you are not interested in receiving personal gifts.

Every organization should set standards of conduct to inform and guide the decision making and conduct of its employees. The standards should be clarified with examples and cases, and they should be regularly discussed among peers and management. To protect the interests of the organization and the reputation of its employees, the standards must be consistently enforced.

Every employee should know the standards for their organization and how those standards affect their own job. When situations arise that your organization's standards do not clearly address, seek advice from a manager. If circumstances do not permit getting advice before you act, ask yourself whether your action, or that of the vendor, might reasonably be misunderstood by another employee or even another vendor. Then, use your best judgment and, afterwards, be certain to disclose your actions to your manager and benefit from his or her own experience and analysis.

CEOs Influencing Hiring Decisions

William A. Nelson, Ph.D.

The organization I lead has an opening in senior management. I know a promising individual whom I would like to bring into the organization for this position, which reports to one of my vice presidents. Am I abusing my authority as CEO by presenting this candidate? How much support can I show for this individual without exerting too much influence on the hiring process?

THE PURPOSE AND challenge of an ethical organization's hiring process are to seek, review, and select appropriate people to fill vacant positions, without bias or prejudice, to help the organization achieve its stated mission. Therefore, while it is acceptable for you, as CEO, to recommend "a promising individual," you must do so carefully.

Like other members of the organization, you should be able to openly recommend candidates for a vacant position. The recommendation should be limited to a simple suggestion, given verbally or in writing, and you should be prepared to answer any questions raised about the candidate during the selection process. Once the recommendation has been made, however, you should limit your involvement in the hiring process to avoid conflicts of interest, or even the appearance of undue influence.

99

The hiring authority should carefully assess your recommended candidate, in the same manner every other candidate is assessed, to determine whether that person possesses the appropriate knowledge, skills, and other attributes necessary to function effectively in the position. Your candidate may turn out to be the best person for the job, in which case he or she should be offered the position. Despite your intentions, the inherent authority of the CEO position can result in an inadvertent conflict of interest if your recommendation is perceived as having greater weight than those of other candidates. You should make clear to the hiring authority that your recommendation is to be treated like all others. This step is absolutely necessary to avoid the perception of a conflict of interest, both by the hiring authority and the rest of the staff.

If the hiring authority believes he or she is expected to blindly hire your candidate, he or she may do so regardless of whether that person is the best for the position. That sends the message to the other candidates for the position, future job candidates, and existing staff that contacts with top management are more important to the organization than a person's skills and qualifications. This would also suggest to these people that ethical standards of impartiality, fairness, and avoidance of conflicts of interest are not valued by you or the organization. Furthermore, hiring a candidate who isn't the most appropriate for the position is unfair to that candidate, the vice president he or she reports to, and the candidate's coworkers.

One of the many roles of the CEO is that of an ethical leader. The CEO's leadership is instrumental in creating an ethical organization through his or her behavior. Therefore, the CEO and the organization's hiring process should function in a manner that reflects, creates, and maintains an ethical environment. CEOs who intentionally or even unintentionally impose their authority on the hiring process ultimately harm themselves and their organizations by eroding their ethical leadership and the ethical nature of the organizations.

Addressing Ethics Accusations

Laurence J. O'Connell Ph.D., S.T.D.

My organization's COO and CFO, both valuable members of my senior management team, are at odds about the advisability of pursuing a costly but potentially worthwhile and profitable new venture. The dispute has escalated to the point that they have made statements to me and other colleagues accusing each other of unethical behavior. What is my ethical responsibility as it relates to exploring their claims and resolving this matter?

AS CEO, YOU are morally and professionally responsible for the ethical character of your organization. Therefore, in making appointments to your senior staff, you should seek candidates who are demonstrably sensitive to ethical issues. Yet, even the most ethically attuned executive staff will encounter ethical conflict and divergent moral opinion.

Moreover, legitimate differences of professional opinion and personal preference are sometimes translated into the language of ethics and mistakenly moved into the realm of moral discourse. It is thus essential to distinguish genuine ethical dissonance from other forms of disagreement and varied perspectives. The following four-step process will allow you to do that by helping you advance ethical insight among your staff, mediate conflicting opinions, and enhance decision making.

Review the facts. Your immediate response to the conflict between the COO and CFO should cut to the heart of the matter. First, you must consider what you believe to be the facts of this situation, then you should talk to the CFO and COO individually to determine how they perceive the facts. Remember that there are no "pure" facts; different people bring different perspectives, resulting in varying viewpoints. Depending on how heated the circumstances have become, you may want to then bring the COO and CFO together to review the facts with you and perhaps reach a shared understanding of the situation.

Identify the ethical values at stake. Ask the COO and CFO what values are at stake and why they have chosen to characterize their disagreement about those values in ethically charged language. Ensure that these executives (as well as the rest of your senior staff) understand that differing opinions, preferences, and motivations do not necessarily constitute an ethical dilemma. Discuss whether these executives have thought through the personal and institutional implications of accusing each other of ethically questionable judgment. Do they know that the use of ethics as a mere rhetorical tool in the absence of a genuine moral dilemma is both dishonest and dangerous, since it easily clouds reason and quickly escalates emotional tensions? If not, you may want to develop a formal framework for ethical analysis to prevent individuals from presuming that an ethical problem exists when it does not or that they enjoy a morally superior position in the face of a problem.

Evaluate the relative weight of conflicting values. As you identify the ethical values at hand, determine how each relates to the others in terms of its importance. This exercise is not intended to determine who is wrong and who is right, but rather show how one legitimate good may have to be sidelined for the sake of another legitimate good to reach a common goal.

Generate a consensus about a morally preferable course of action that is consistent with your organization's mission and values. By doing this, you can take the disagreement out of the subjective, personal arena and put it in the context of your organization's goals.

Unless egregious unethical behavior is in the immediate offing, the conflict between the COO and CFO represents a teachable moment for the entire senior staff. In the face of such a situation, be sure to use this opportunity to evaluate how genuine ethical problems are detected, acknowledged, and handled maturely within your organization.

ACHE's Ethics Self-Assessment Instrument is useful [see Appendix C] for evaluating your responses to ethical dilemmas.

Reporting Unethical Behavior

John Abbott Worthley, D.P.A.

I have recently accepted a position with a new organization. One of the reasons I'm leaving my current organization is because I believe my supervisor has, on a number of occasions, made unethical decisions. What is my responsibility to make my concerns known before I leave?

THE QUESTION OF responsibility that you raise is ever timely and terribly important. Almost all of us, at some time in our careers, will be privy to things that seem untoward in our workplace. At these times, is it ethical to just walk away, leaving our unit or organization in a continuing questionable situation when, indeed, we could do something?

On the other hand, is it ethical to just blow the whistle and potentially destroy a fellow professional and harm an otherwise good healthcare organization?

In addressing these questions, the issues of judgment and accountability are key. First, you need to determine whose judgment of whether behavior is "unethical" is appropriate and what organizational accountability mechanisms are in place to deal with questionable situations.

When difficult decisions are made, and you disagree with them, those decisions can appear to you to be unethical while, at the same time, appear ethical to others. Whose judgment should prevail? If the behavior clearly violates a legal statute or a code of ethics, that is one thing; but if individuals simply have different opinions of what is "right," that may be another matter. Furthermore, when one of those individuals is in a position of legitimate authority, the question of whose judgment should prevail is all the more salient.

Second, formal accountability mechanisms, such as ethics committees, legal offices, grievance procedures, and professional associations, are often in place and can be quite helpful in handling such a situation. In addition, many informal accountability mechanisms, such as discussions with colleagues and the supervisor involved, are also available. If you have not discussed your concerns with the supervisor, for example, the questions of ethical fairness and respect could be raised.

Third, you must consider the consequences of the various options. You could, of course, just go on to the new job and leave it at that. You would suffer no repercussions, but your former organization, colleagues, and clients or patients would continue in the questionable situation.

If your organization has a formal ethics review procedure, you could pursue that avenue, either openly or perhaps anonymously. Reporting the situation to a superior within the organization is an option that can keep the matter more confidential, but it could cause problems for you or that superior.

Reporting the supervisor to an external authority would probably bring corrective action but could affect the organization's reputation as well as your own. Discussing your concerns with the supervisor could have a wide range of consequences, depending on the individual.

Before taking action, you may want to discuss the problem with a discreet third party, such as a friend from another division or company. It can help you gain some perspective and avoid hasty decisions, and prevent you from falling into arbitrariness and self-righteousness.

Overall, if your supervisor's behavior is a clear violation of an articulated ethical standard, your responsibility is more evident. If, on the other hand, it is a situation of some ethical ambiguity, you need to carefully consider the individual circumstances, issues, and people involved to discern the ethically mature response.

Rumors of Unethical Conduct

Gary Edwards, J.D.

*I am the CEO of a healthcare organization that has CEOs from local busi-
nesses serving on its board. Lately, I have heard rumors that one CEO is
involved in some unethical business practices at his own organization. I
don't know if the rumors are true, and this person has always been a
valuable member of my board, but I am afraid of damage to my organization's reputation if the rumors become widely known. What are my responsibilities to my organization and to this board member?*

AS AN OFFICER and, presumably, director of your organization,
your obligation to protect the interests of the organization, its owners, and the community outweighs any individual consideration
you may have for your board member. That said, questions still remain. Chief among them is whether the rumors are true, what you
should do to determine that, and what actions you should take if
you find the rumors accurate.

Even if unfounded, rumors of grossly unethical business practices by an organization's CEO will certainly harm that individual's
own reputation and may well cost the organization the business of
those who believe the rumors to be true. The damage to your own
organization will depend, in part, on the nature of the misconduct
that is rumored.

Some actions (such as improperly disclosing confidential information of one supplier to another) will likely damage the board member's organization, but may not reflect on or harm your own. Under such circumstances, you might not be obliged to investigate the rumors, but you might wish to advise your board member of what you have heard. The board member could then correct erroneous rumors or, if they were true, correct his or her practices and possibly make amends.

However, other types of rumors might pose significant risks for your own organization. For instance, if the purported misconduct concerned insider trading or the improper gathering and use of competitive intelligence, you should certainly be concerned for your organization's reputation. Additionally, you must consider that, if the rumors are true, your organization might have been similarly victimized by the board member. Under some circumstances, your organization might not be directly at risk, but you might nevertheless be obliged to take action to prevent harm to the public or to disclose ongoing criminal activities.

For example, if the rumors concerned alleged illegal conduct, you might wish to advise legal or regulatory authorities of the rumored activities.

The exact activities that are alleged and the source of those allegations dictate what specific actions you should take. However, here are a few general suggestions for handling these rumors of unethical conduct:

1. Get legal advice before responding to the rumored misconduct.
2. Consistent with the obligations and constraints of that advice, limit the spread of the rumors by not repeating them yourself.
3. Initiate or implement appropriate action to protect the public, your organization, and, if possible, your board member's reputation. Depending on the particular facts and circumstances, this may be as simple as informing your board member of the

rumors about his or her business practices, or it may involve advising your board of directors, his or her organization's board, or legal and regulatory authorities.

Dealing with rumors of misconduct is always challenging, as your obligations often conflict with one another. In this case, your primary duty is to your organization; however, beware of acting on rumors before you are certain of their accuracy.

Trust and Physician Payment

Susan Dorr Goold, M.D.

As the healthcare organization I work for has grown, it has developed different types of relationships with physicians: some are employed and some belong to independent physician groups. Additionally, the physicians participate in a variety of managed care plans. As a result, physicians are paid differently for the same procedures depending on the type of relationship they have with the organization or the different plans. What are the ethical implications of this?

DIFFERENCES IN HEALTHCARE reimbursement can certainly influence a patient's experience of care. These differences can also potentially affect the physician-patient relationship, which is fiduciary and trust-based—that is, it is characterized by a power imbalance, a vulnerability on the part of the patient, and social and legal expectations that the physician will act in the patient's best interests.

Managed care has been criticized for paying physicians in ways that could undermine this relationship by creating a conflict between the interest of the patient and the financial interest of the physician. However, all ways in which physicians are paid have the potential to influence decision making and patient experiences of care. Capitation, risk withholds, or large bonuses that depend on utilization measures can create an incentive for physicians to provide fewer rather than more services. Fee-for-service reimbursement can create incentives to provide more rather than fewer services, and salaried arrangements can affect physician productivity and the willingness to see patients urgently. All of these are potential conflicts of interest to some degree.

The question is, which payment mechanisms create conflicts of interests that are *unduly intrusive* into the physician-patient relationship and individual clinical decision making? It depends on the type of incentive and the extent to which its impact is diffused. Risk withholds, for instance, in which referrals or tests are paid for out of a pool and the unspent remainder returned to the physician, are tightly linked to individual patient decisions. So are fee-for-service payments. In contrast, diffusing financial risk over a large number of physicians or patients weakens the link between income and a single clinical decision. Similarly, multiple payment mechanisms will prevent one payer's reimbursement from causing an unduly intrusive conflict of interest in individual clinical decisions.

Besides the intrusion into physician-patient decision making, certain financial incentives have another effect—on the perceptions of patients. Trust is vulnerable to such perceptions and can be undermined if patients or members of a health plan believe, correctly or incorrectly, that their physicians do not have the best interests of patients at heart. Consider the following examples:

- A physician in a fee-for-service system receives $60 for a 15-minute office visit. In the same system, a physician could receive $1,500 for a 20-minute procedure. In both cases, the link between physician income and a single clinical decision is tight. This can be an incentive to overuse services—a conflict of interest that could lead patients to distrust their physicians. In addition, the incentive is potentially more intrusive when the dollar amount is large.

- A small physician practice is capitated for a small number of patients. Concern with economic survival and an inability to spread risk make the incentive to alter individual decisions on the basis of economic interest unduly intrusive. Consider in contrast, a large, multispecialty group practice that is capitated for a large population of patients and has multiple payers, some of whom reimburse through noncapitated mechanisms. In this case, the capitation influences the group as a whole more than individual physicians; the ability to diffuse risk also weakens the link between income and single patient care decisions. The payment mechanism in this case does not intrude unduly into the decision or the physician-patient relationship.

- A risk withhold system in which payment for referrals, x-rays, and other services come out of the physicians' potential bonus pool can be a strong incentive that is linked tightly to individual decisions. In effect, the physician loses money whenever he or she refers a patient or orders an expensive test, and this could intrude consciously or subconsciously into individual patient care decisions. In addition, patients who are aware of this means of reimbursement may second-guess their physician's advice.

Research suggests that better health outcomes are linked to strong physician-patient relationships. In contrast, relationships characterized by a lack of trust can lead to unnecessary use of services as patients request or demand them. Maintaining the trust of your patients is not only an ethical and clinical imperative, it is a matter of your organization's long-term survival.

Changes in physician reimbursement may help promote prudent use of limited healthcare resources. However, they can also drastically or subtly weaken the fiduciary, trust-based relationship that is a cornerstone of healthcare. This is not restricted to prepaid capitated systems or managed care plans—all reimbursement types can be intrusive, or at least appear to be. As a healthcare executive, it is crucial that you critically scrutinize the ways in which your individual physicians are reimbursed by your organization, their group practice, or outside health plans, and ensure that those payment mechanisms do not damage patient trust by appearing to intrude unduly into physicians' decision making.

PART VII

Clinical Ethics Issues

Increased Protection
of Patient Rights

David C. Thomasma, Ph.D.

THE JOINT COMMISSION issued new guidelines for accreditation of hospitals in its *Accreditation Manual for Hospitals*. The Joint Commission's new standards for protecting patient rights will have a major impact on the ethical duties of healthcare managers, the way the Joint Commission will conduct its reviews, and the role of all staff—especially nurses—in resolving ethical dilemmas. In addition, greater professional demands will be placed on ethics committees and ethics consult services.

First, the Joint Commission's standards emphasize that institutions must have mechanisms for resolving ethical dilemmas. Through the Patient Self-Determination Act, an institution's response to a patient's rights and treatment decisions will be monitored for effectiveness. Indeed, healthcare administration will be held accountable for the ethical behavior of the healthcare organization. Appropriate mechanisms are left to each institution, but they must function well. For most institutions, an ethics committee will be the mechanism of choice.

Second, the Joint Commission will augment its chart reviews through interviews with key staff and patients. Questions will most likely concern the quality and effectiveness of the ethical resolution mechanisms. Do patients know that the ethics committee or alternate procedures exist? Does the staff? How is access provided? What are the objectives of this service? Does it include an ethics consult service? How are dilemmas resolved?

Third, the Joint Commission pays special attention to the nurse's role in resolving ethical dilemmas. For too long, nurses have felt like second-class citizens in this process, even though they have often spearheaded institutional efforts to establish and maintain hospital ethics committees. Most likely, a greater focus on ethics education for nursing staff will be a direct result of this Joint Commission interest. To a greater extent than in the past, the ethics committee should be involved with such educational efforts.

Finally, the role of the ethics committee will be more professionalized by the Joint Commission's underlining of ethical duties of healthcare organizations. In the first place, ethics committees most often were established to promote dialogue about ethical dilemmas and make recommendations about guidelines or policies such as "do not resuscitate orders." Some of the more established committees are entering a midlife crisis now that initial work has been accomplished. The Joint Commission has changed all that. Charged with protecting a patient's rights and autonomy, the ethics committee will enter the mainstream of guiding the institution's commitments and mission.

The ethics committee will be evaluated, not only by the Joint Commission, but also by the institution itself, by staff, and by patients. This will cause the ethics committee to become more aware of its role and function within the institution, and rectify its shortcomings through better education and procedures. In addition, training and certification of the consult service, if it is provided for specific case dilemmas, will most certainly be developed. Among ethics consultants this process is currently being hotly debated. It is an idea whose time has come.

Kudos to the Joint Commission for its support of mechanisms for resolving ethical dilemmas in healthcare organizations.

Institutional Advance Directives

David C. Thomasma, Ph.D.

THE PATIENT SELF-DETERMINATION Act (PSDA) is worth celebrating because it continues to raise the awareness of health-care workers, patients, and the community about the rights of individuals to express their wishes about life-and-death medical decisions. It also opens the door to a whole new set of issues about an organization's advance directives.

Since patients are always vulnerable within the context of institutional healthcare delivery, it is the responsibility of healthcare institutions to ensure that informed consent be at its premium in all activities surrounding intervention and care. In this regard, is it sufficient to ensure proper procedures for the PSDA? Perhaps not.

Only about 10 percent of patients are taking advantage of the opportunity to develop their advance directives prior to their admission in healthcare institutions. While this is a major advance over the minuscule number choosing to do so in the past, it still leaves a lot to be desired.

What happens if patients do not choose to exercise their right to execute an advance directive?

For one thing, both the patient and the institution become vulnerable in the future to interventions that may not be foreseen at present, and that may violate the person's values or the institution's ability to survive by reason of an overload of uncompensated care. Both the patient and institution may wind up in a bottomless pit of healthcare.

Defining the nature of care within the institution in the absence of patient wishes or directives is an important part of acting circumspectly and prudently managing our resources. This approach is also a matter of justice—treating all persons fairly and equitably without providing excessive care for one patient to the detriment of others who cannot even obtain basic care.

As we gain more familiarity and experience with the PSDA, objective, scientific studies need to be made about choices people made when given the opportunity to think about the consequences of intervention before a crisis actually occurred. These objective measures of choices might then be used by healthcare institutions to help interpret the standards of care and the limits of care that might guide caregivers in the absence of advance directives on the part of patients. Such guides, of course, would insufficiently protect vulnerable patients from harm, without an advance declaration on the part of the institution itself.

Thus, when patients decline the invitation to exercise their right to tell caregivers in advance of their wishes, for whatever reason, the next step in the dialogue might be a list of care interventions that can be implemented, and those that may not be, on the part of the institution. The patient and family would then know in advance what the standards of care for various illnesses would be at a particular healthcare facility. Sometimes these standards of care might be advertised. At the very least they could become part of the more detailed package defining the institution's mission and philosophy.

These standards of care, in the absence of advance directives, would constitute institutional advance directives. This may be the next logical step in improving informed consent, the just distribution of goods and services in our society, and protecting institutions from offering medically useless therapy.

The Executive's Role
in Clinical Matters

Paul B. Hofmann, Dr.P.H., FACHE

IT IS NOT surprising that healthcare executives are more comfortable dealing with financial rather than medical reports. After all, the governing board and management staff has a well-established fiduciary responsibility to make prudent decisions in allocating an organization's limited resources. But in a healthcare organization, the role of senior executives should not be limited to management issues. Healthcare executives must establish a role in clinical matters as well.

Many believe that clinical subjects are largely the prerogative of formally trained professionals such as physicians, nurses, pharmacists, social workers, therapists, and others. Some even suggest that executives should not play a role in influencing clinical decisions. These observers view direct involvement as infringing on the authority of the professional staff. Furthermore, intervention by executives who lack clinical credentials could be considered hazardous to their job security. The clinical activity of healthcare executives, according to this perspective, should be restricted to supporting the recruitment and retention of the best qualified staff available and being responsive to legitimate requests for essential resources.

Given the prevailing arguments, why should executives assert themselves in clinical matters and what actions are reasonable? The answer to the first question is inescapable: They should not abdicate total responsibility for such a fundamental organizational function, namely the provision of the highest possible quality patient care. Executives have a moral obligation to be involved in these matters and can do so without detracting from or interfering with the role of clinical chiefs of service, medical staff officers, or the medical director/vice president of medical affairs.

Depending on the size and complexity of the organization, it may be unrealistic for senior executives to be knowledgeable about every unusual development affecting specific patients and physicians. Nonetheless, an increase in litigation cases should certainly not be what alerts the management staff to a potential pattern of poor-quality care. For example, regardless of a change in the number of formal legal claims, executives should be familiar with the results of quality assurance and risk management reports.

To demonstrate a genuine sensitivity for clinical issues, senior administrative staff members should make routine patient rounds. In addition to the value of interacting directly with patients and their families and receiving candid, timely assessments of patient care, this activity creates a natural opportunity to communicate with physicians, nurses, and other staff.

Whether the setting is an acute care floor, skilled nursing care facility, or a home care residence, making patient rounds permits the executive to obtain firsthand knowledge about what influences clinical decisions. Moreover, the mere physical presence of the executive conveys a personal interest in and concern about both the people receiving care and those furnishing it.

Periodic, if not regular, attendance at medical staff grand rounds and meetings of the organization's ethics committee can also help executives remain aware of current clinical developments and their implications. This type of involvement contributes to the executive's continuing education. In addition, it allows for more informed decision making when executives allocate organizational resources.

By strengthening their involvement in clinical matters, healthcare executives are better able to lead their organizations in providing high-quality patient care.

Making Life-Ending Decisions

Sister Irene Kraus, LFACHE

Recently my organization expended considerable resources to treat a 30-year-old woman whose condition was deemed futile. Despite the care we provided and the resources we expended, she died within 12 hours of admission. In such situations, when resources are scarce, how can we determine when enough has been done?

THE DILEMMA OF the question being posed is: Are we prolonging life beyond what was and is considered morally and humanly acceptable?

For decades, no one wanted to talk about death and dying. It was looked on as a fact of life no one wanted to face. Then came the boom in medical technology, which has allowed medical caregivers to actualize events that were once only dreams. Perhaps our technological progress has backfired on us.

From the ashes have risen new terms and new concepts such as the "right to die." Is there truly such a thing? We have no choice whether we want to die. It's inevitable that we will. Of all the creatures on the face of the earth, only the human species is aware that it is dying. As a result, it would seem that we must make this event in our lives as sacred as possible. Nevertheless, that does not mean that we must use everything known to the medical profession to prolong life.

Families and caregivers must have norms to guide life-ending decisions. A balance must be struck between use of extraordinary means and costly procedures and the dignity of the patient, and the latter cannot be compromised. The decision to withhold or discontinue extraordinary or disproportionate means of medical intervention must be made with the judgment that the treatment itself is excessively burdensome or that the treatment is useless. It should never be made on the basis that the person's life is not worth living.

One ethicist, Elena Muller-Garcia, offered this advice: "Answering the following questions will help to determine when a treatment may be withheld or withdrawn:

- Is it too painful?
- Is it too physically damaging?
- Is it psychologically repugnant to the patient?
- Does it suppress too greatly the patient's mental capacity?
- Is the expense prohibitive?

If the answer to all of these questions is 'yes,' the extraordinary treatment may be withdrawn."

Sometimes families or caregivers are concerned that a course of treatment may be "useless" or "burdensome." This issue can only be addressed on an individual basis since what is useless to one person might not be useless to another. For example, what might be considered appropriate treatment for a 30-year old who is terminally ill might be completely inappropriate for an 80-year old. Aside from age, other possible norms might be whether the treatment brings about the effect for which it was designed (if not, it is medically inappropriate), the condition of the patient, and the benefit to be derived from the treatment.

Finally, patient concerns must be addressed regarding the decision whether to withhold life-sustaining treatment. I encourage everyone to have a living will; to have in writing what his or her desires might be relative to the established norms; to have a health "guardian" in the event that one cannot decide for oneself; and to have a dialogue with one's family, clergyman, and physicians before a life-and-death crisis occurs. [See Appendix B5 for ACHE's Ethical Policy Statement "Decisions Near the End of Life"].

Ensuring Compliance
with Advance Directives

Mark H. Waymack, Ph.D.

As a hospital CEO, *I have made sure we are in compliance with the Patient Self-Determination Act. However, it has come to my attention that one member of our medical staff has a history of not abiding by patients' advance directives. What is my responsibility as* CEO *to balance respect for patients' directives with respect for physicians' autonomy?*

AN INCREASED RESPECT for patient self-determination has been one of healthcare ethics' most emphasized goals during the last 20 years. Advance directives extend patients' self-determination into situations where individuals can no longer speak for themselves. A medical institution has a moral obligation, further reinforced by federal legislation to follow those directives.

The role of CEO includes responsibility for moral leadership, but it is surely neither prudent nor efficient to try to micromanage the ethics of the organization. Rather, it would be far better to take the actions of the individual physician as a symptom of a potential systemic problem.

This case, centering on a physician's persistent practice of ignoring or finding ways to override patients' advance directives, raises several issues. First, advance directives remain far less effective in promoting patient self-determination than ethicists and legislators might have wished. Only a small fraction of people ever execute advance directives, and even in cases where such directives do exist, patients' expressed wishes are often overruled by physicians or family members. If the CEO approaches this issue as a social or cultural problem, he or she can address it by encouraging greater efforts to educate the medical staff on ethical issues surrounding advance directives.

Such efforts, however, may seem remote from the particular question at hand, which is: What should the CEO do about this particular physician's pattern of disobeying advance directives? To address this particular issue, it would help to know how this problem was brought to the CEO's attention. Did it come by way of the grapevine or through formal networks, such as the ethics committee or the chief of staff? The distinction is important because the CEO must walk a fine line between exerting moral leadership for the organization and interfering in a physician's professional decision making.

If the CEO learned of the problem through the grapevine, the managerial cost of intervening in a physician practice issue, uninvited by the medical staff, could be quite high. Physicians, after all, are professionals who possess special knowledge and, consequently, a measure of professional autonomy. To second-guess a physician's judgment, even in egregious cases, sets a precedent of administrative interference that other physicians would most likely view with deep mistrust.

So, as CEO, what is one to do? This brings us to another element of the ethical problem: What sort of ethical issues in management does this case present?

First, this CEO must examine the institution's ethics mechanisms to determine whether they are sufficient to handle this and other similar problems. If so, the CEO must ensure that all ethical conflicts are addressed within these standard procedures. If not, the

CEO's most appropriate and effective course of action would be to reexamine the structure and position of the ethics committee, identifying ways to expand its educational efforts and strengthen its position within the institution. The CEO should encourage everyone in the institution to see the ethics committee as a useful resource for addressing and preventing problems such as this one.

The CEO has a managerial responsibility to provide moral leadership for the organization. While one might quibble about particular cases, it is clearly unethical to support a practice pattern of violating patient self-determination. So the question becomes not so much what to do about an individual physician's actions, but rather how to lead the organization so that the risks of any physician habitually violating patient advance directives is minimized.

Dealing with Noncompliant Patients

Paul B. Hofmann, Dr.P.H., FACHE

We have a dialysis patient, with a history of mental illness, who periodically insists that treatment be discontinued. Often, this patient becomes verbally abusive and disruptive if treatment is not stopped. Is it ethically justified to force a patient to accept treatment?

REGARDLESS OF THEIR mental status, patients will often decline treatment or insist that it be discontinued. As people become better educated about issues related to their care and more assertive in expressing their preferences, healthcare facilities should recognize that refusal to accept recommended therapy might become more common. To address these situations, healthcare organizations should develop noncompliant patient policies.

REASONS FOR DEVELOPING A POLICY ON NONCOMPLIANT PATIENTS

Each case will present its own unique set of circumstances, but handling every incident on an ad hoc basis will serve neither the patient's nor your organization's best interests. For at least three reasons, you should develop a policy on noncompliant patients before you need to apply it:

1. It is always preferable to create a policy in a noncrisis mode since myriad issues must be considered in dealing with noncompliant patients. The document should be prepared, reviewed, and refined in a time frame not compressed by the urgency associated with a specific situation.
2. A carefully constructed policy will always include input from your organization's attorney. Compelling a patient to accept treatment or alternatively, withholding or discontinuing treatment, could have obvious legal consequences. Certainly, you want to fully explore these issues before an evening or weekend telephone call to your on-call administrator.
3. A comprehensive policy provides direction and support to your staff and increases the likelihood that patients and their families are treated consistently. Healthcare professionals—including physicians, nurses, and social workers—are often morally stressed by noncompliant patients. As noted below, an effective policy will recognize that not only do patients have rights, but so does your staff.

ELEMENTS OF A NONCOMPLIANT PATIENT POLICY

Although the actual content of an organization's policy will vary—reflecting individual missions, values, and cultures—each policy should have common elements:

Preface. This general introduction should describe your policy's purpose. For example, it should acknowledge that patients and their surrogate decision makers may not comply with diagnostic or treatment plans. In such instances, steps should be taken to preserve their rights and responsibilities, as well as those of staff. The comfort and safety of other patients must also be protected.

Definition of noncompliance. A patient may be verbally abusive, physically combative, or exhibit other behavior that makes it difficult and perhaps impossible to perform diagnostic or therapeutic procedures. Clarifying how patients are deemed "noncompliant" will help determine appropriate responses. Responses should vary depending on whether the conduct will irreversibly compromise the patient's clinical condition. The relative risks and benefits of intervention and nonintervention must be weighed. A distinction should be made between patients who exercise the right of autonomy via relatively "benign" noncompliance (refusal to eat a meal) and patients whose behavior significantly compromises others or whose level of nonadherence to a medical plan makes that plan futile.

Determination of decision-making capacity. A patient could be legally incompetent to make an informed decision about his or her care—perhaps because of age, in the case of a minor, or as the result of medication, trauma, or disease. In the latter circumstances, patients can move in and out of decision-making capacity, so caution must be exercised to preserve their right to make an informed consent or refusal when justified. Options for assessing mental competency should be described.

Assurance of continuity of care. Regardless of a patient's aberrant behavior, your organization has a responsibility to maintain continuity of care. For example, you may need to arrange the patient's transfer to another unit within your organization or to a more suitable organization elsewhere. The policy should stipulate who has the primary role to explore and coordinate these arrangements.

Promotion of patient rights and responsibilities. In addition to having the right to make an informed consent or refusal and to receive continuity of care, patients have other rights as well as responsibilities. These should be covered in a separate document on this topic, and it can simply be referenced in the policy or provided as an addendum.

Recognition of staff rights and responsibilities. When employees believe their physical safety is being compromised, or verbal harassment has become intolerable, a procedure should be available so they can request prompt assistance with the immediate problem. This section of the policy should describe how a long-term solution will be provided if the relief is only temporary and the problem continues. It should also delineate your staff's responsibilities for addressing the needs of noncompliant patients.

Description of available resources. In addition to legal counsel, the potential role of your organization's risk manager, ethics committee, chaplaincy service, and other resources in dealing with a noncompliant patient should be explained.

Summary of procedure. The policy should describe the sequence of activities necessary to achieve timely closure to the case. For example, first, be sure to document pertinent issues and discussions in the patient's medical record. Next, you many find it helpful to make a contract with noncompliant patients, describing expectations and related contingencies should inappropriate behavior continue. The responsible healthcare provider should also meet with the patient and, where appropriate, the patient's family (or others with a significant role in the patient's life) to discuss the consequences of continued noncompliant behavior before discontinuing care to an abusive, threatening, or uncooperative patient. Furthermore, you may want to delineate the use and content of a preliminary letter of warning and, if necessary, the use and content of a dismissal letter in your policy. Finally, there must be acknowledgment of the requirement, under federal law, to provide emergency care.

A RESPONSE TO THE DIALYSIS CASE

Forcing a patient to accept treatment under specific circumstances is ethically justified. Such circumstances would include a patient who:

- is diagnosed with a life-threatening clinical condition;
- is a minor or legally incompetent because of illness or trauma;
- does not have an advanced directive that contraindicates intervention; or
- has a legally empowered surrogate who authorizes treatment.

Before taking any action, you should thoroughly review existing facts and collect missing information to ensure a comprehensive assessment of the issues and alternative actions. The safety of other patients and staff must not be jeopardized. You must also proceed in a manner that will avoid charges of abandonment or discrimination if services are terminated. The availability of a comprehensive policy on noncompliant patients, reflecting your organization's mission, culture, and values, should help create an ethical and appropriate response to these situations.

The Ethical and Legal Imperatives of Medical Errors

E. Haavi Morreim, Ph.D.

In addition to the highly publicized Institute of Medicine report about the prevalence of medical errors, a number of other studies have brought greater attention to this issue. Acknowledging that traditional risk management programs are important but not sufficient, how can my organization respond to the ethical and legal imperatives to be more successful in reducing medical errors?

AN ERROR, ACCORDING to the Institute of Medicine, is either a mistake in execution (the correct action did not proceed as intended) or a problem of planning (the intended action itself was not correct). Errors are not to be confused with risks or side effects, whose incidence is known but whose occurrence is not avoidable. To address the issues surrounding errors, we must distinguish ethical from legal imperatives.

ETHICAL IMPERATIVES

There are two major ethical imperatives: 1) avoid errors wherever possible and, when they do occur, 2) do right by the people who are

141

harmed. For avoiding errors, excellent ideas are now emerging, such as bar code drug delivery systems, integrated computer information systems, and blame-free error reporting followed by root cause analysis. Organizations should seek real and continuing improvement, not just window dressing.

Doing the right thing when an error occurs requires a broad view because patients are not the only ones who may be harmed. Physicians and other providers may be emotionally devastated in a medical culture that emphasizes perfection, self-reproach, and go-it-alone responsibility. When the error stems from ordinary human failings like fatigue, physicians' guilt may be undeserved; nevertheless it can impede their effectiveness in caring for patients in the future, as well as their willingness to participate in error-reduction efforts. Organizations need to help all staff cope effectively with those responses.

Where an avoidable error has led to significant harm or death, doing right by patients and families is, of course, the primary focus. Patients and families need to be told what happened, kept abreast of the investigation, and informed about efforts to prevent recurrences. Healthcare organizations should also offer reasonable compensation that will place those who are injured as close as possible to the position they would have been in had the error not occurred.

Not only is this the fair thing to do, but providing such information and assistance can yield two further benefits. First, only if patients and families know about the error can they provide additional information to assist in a root cause analysis that, in turn, might help prevent similar errors. Second, every risk manager has heard patients and families insist that "this must never happen to anyone else." Participation in the organization's improvement process can help those who have suffered from error to find personal value and meaning in a tragic situation.

The ethical imperative to help restore patients and families as close as possible to their "pre-error" state has the ring of tort law because, in this area, good ethics is also good law. The essence of fault-based tort law is not to extract money from the richest person. Rather, it is to make sure that innocent people do not have to bear the costs when they are injured by another's carelessness. Conversely, if no one is specifically at fault, then shifting the blame for the misfortune on organizations or individuals simply because they have "deep pockets" is equally unfair.

That is the ideal, at any rate. Today's judicial realities, however, do not always match this ideal. Courts are sometimes quick to find "fault" in the actions of whichever party has the money to help an injured patient.

There is nothing inherently wrong with prudent self-interest, although it should take a backseat to important ethical mandates. Fortunately, in this area there may not be as much conflict as organizations assume. *Annals of Internal Medicine* recently reported that one hospital's experience with "extreme honesty" was economically as well as ethically superior. After a single year in which two judgments alone cost $1.5 million, a Kentucky VA hospital began investigating errors thoroughly; informing patients and families when errors had caused injury or death; helping them to find legal representation; and then negotiating a mutually agreeable arrangement for restitution, compensation, and/or corrective action. After seven years under this new policy, the hospital's payouts for settlements and malpractice claims totaled only $1.3 million.

A flurry of studies over the past decade suggests that people often sue for reasons having little to do with medical negligence or even adverse outcomes. Rather, suits are commonly filed because of anger and poor relationships. In one study, 48 percent of mothers of dead or injured infants felt that the physician had actually tried to mislead them, and 70 percent felt that the physician had not warned them adequately regarding the infant's long-term problems. And many patients sue when they conclude that filing a claim is the only way to find out what really happened.

In the end, error reduction, combined with appropriate disclosure and compensation, appears to offer abundant opportunities in which good ethics is also good healthcare and good business.

PART VIII

Organizational Ethics Issues

Access to Healthcare

David C. Thomasma, Ph.D.

A NATIONAL CONSENSUS is building for reform of the health-care system. This movement comes with good reason. Virtually alone among advanced countries, the United States does not yet consider it a right for all citizens to have equal access to healthcare. At the very least, basic healthcare coverage for all is a desirable goal. It is not just unfortunate that millions of us have no access to healthcare and that the middle class often can no longer afford it. Rather, it is unjust since not providing it has been an act of political will.

Reform stems from two competing interests. Some support for reform arises from high-minded principles of justice while other support stems from a desire to control costs that rise annually at twice the rate of inflation. Many countries have been able to combine both interests, but it is difficult. How can we simultaneously provide greater coverage at less cost? The issue was confined to academic discussion until voters voiced their concerns. Presidential candidates are now touting their own vision of such reform, as are members of Congress. In the midst of the politics, it is too easy to forget that healthcare is a good and a service prerequisite for the well-being of all human beings.

In earlier times, the essential moral quality of healthcare was embedded in the professional codes of the caregivers. With the rise of modern, technological healthcare, the former one-on-one relationship between doctor and patient became institutionalized. Hospitals were no longer like a hotel where physicians signed patients in and out at will. Suddenly, with escalating costs and subsequent social and political monitoring, the doctor-patient relation became one with third-party payers and institutions.

There are some overriding ethical considerations in the design of any national health program. First, patients should have control over their care so that they do not experience difficulties and delays in obtaining appropriate and approved treatment. Second, the moral character of the institutions of health delivery and the practitioners of healthcare must not be destroyed by bureaucratic requirements. Third, since some form of rationing will be required regarding specific treatments to be made available, the national health program should be as efficient as possible. This means greater effort must be made to put available monies in patient care rather than in administrative overhead costs. Fourth, the quality of human judgment and flexibility for treating individual differences should be maintained as far as possible so formulaic responses to human pain and misery are avoided.

Incentives to hold down costs and to increase the quality of care should be built into the plan. But so too should incentives to cooperate rather than compete to ensure commitment to patients and their values as well as the survival of institutions. No institution should benefit by shunning essential care. A plan for sharing the burden of expensive and unreimbursed care among institutions should be incorporated into the national health program.

Healthcare institutions can be said to have a "conscience." This is a convenient shorthand for the sum total of their mission and commitments. Individuals within institutions, including the physicians practicing there, should have a say in the formation of the institution's mission and values and should commit to them. If healthcare executives try to arrange for the care of individuals without healthcare insurance, then physicians with admitting privileges might be asked to help. If they refuse, should they be allowed to continue to have such privileges if their refusal violates a commitment of the institution and its leaders and staff?

Ethics and the Governing Board

Robert E. Toomey, LL.D., LFACHE

WHILE IT IS management's responsibility to ensure that the healthcare organization is fulfilling its ethical responsibility to patients, their families, the community, and staff, monitoring the ethical heartbeat of the healthcare organization is clearly a board responsibility, too.

For the board and management to appropriately lead the organization in fulfilling its mission, an ethical framework for policymaking must be available and routinely applied. To create that framework, the board and management must establish an ethical imperative.

For organizations owned and operated by a recognized religious group, establishing an ethical foundation is a relatively simple matter because policymaking is rooted in the religious beliefs of its owners. Creating this ethical framework in other healthcare organizations requires specific efforts. Although not founded on religious principles, these organizations were established out of dedication to community. It is on this principle that these organizations must build.

Often healthcare leaders view ethics in terms of medical care, but they also must look at ethics in terms of operations. They must ensure that organizational ethics uphold moral standards and emphasize the delivery of high-quality service and care.

At the board level, policies must be developed to promote the delivery of high-quality service and care as well as enhance the well-being of the organization. Policies must be created and established that will enable the organization to achieve its vision in an equitable and rational manner.

In the face of a rapidly changing healthcare environment and the changing needs of those the organization serves, it is critical for the board and management staff to periodically re-evaluate their organizations' existing ethical frameworks. To assess your organization's ethical foundation, ask yourself the following questions:

- Are our organization's services meeting community needs?
- Are acquisitions and our use of financial resources consistent with our organization's overall mission?
- Are we creating and designing facilities to address community needs?
- Is our organization providing high-quality care, and are adequate physician resources and appropriate medical care available to meet community needs?
- Are we fulfilling our role in educating the community, patients, physicians, employees, and others as needed?
- Are we making available the human resources, supplies, and equipment necessary to provide high-quality services to our patients?
- What have we done to develop stronger relations with the community and all other key stakeholders?

ORGANIZATIONAL VALUES

Decisions that can be evaluated against and found consistent with organizational values will demonstrate the moral and ethical strength of the organization. The healthcare organization has a soul and a spirit, a personality and a culture. Today's healthcare leaders must thoroughly understand that their actions can strengthen or weaken the ethical fibers of their organization.

Ethics and the Business of Healthcare

Thomas C. Dolan, Ph.D., FACHE, CAE

WE HAVE WITNESSED a transformation in the way healthcare services are financed and delivered in the past few years. With the growth of managed care, the emergence of large nationwide healthcare systems, and rapid advances in medical technology, the business of healthcare delivery—and our responsibility for managing it—has changed. Despite the many unknowns we now face, healthcare executives are expected to continue to take action and make decisions about healthcare delivery on a daily basis. The changes in the field, and the choices they are forcing us to make, however, are posing increasingly complicated ethical questions.

I was given the opportunity to join 44 physicians, nurses, healthcare executives, ethicists, academic policy analysts, and religious leaders at the Woodstock Seminar in Business Ethics to discuss some of the ethical dilemmas now facing healthcare providers. Sponsored by the Woodstock Theological Center at Georgetown University, the seminar spanned two years and consisted of four conferences where we explored the question, "What are the most pressing ethical issues healthcare providers face?"

Through intense discussion, we identified a number of common ethical dilemmas, including:

- Meeting patient needs with scarce resources
- Providing the most appropriate care when providers profit from patient use of specific resources or when rules and regulations conflict with professional judgment
- Acting in the best interest of the patient when reporting requirements may be in conflict with patient confidentiality
- Making appropriate care decisions when patients' behaviors contribute significantly to their problems
- Appropriately using new or unproven technologies

The debate on these issues was heated, and while it was impossible to reach consensus on the "most appropriate" behavior in each situation, the discussion was enlightening, providing us with an opportunity to honestly assess the implications of various scenarios on patients and providers. Through these discussions, we decided that while not everyone will act alike, all healthcare providers are obligated to make decisions within a basic ethical framework built on compassion and respect for human dignity, commitment to professional competence, spirit of service, honesty, confidentiality, good stewardship, and careful administration.

OTHER FINDINGS

As another part of our discussions, we developed a checklist of questions healthcare executives can ask as they address the dilemmas cited above. While not exhaustive, the following examples will give you a feel for the quality of our discussions:

- Have I made a sincere effort to determine the needs and resources in my community and arrive at a principled estimate of my institution's fair share of uncompensated care?
- Do I believe a preferred treatment is important enough to the health of the patient that I would recommend it if the patient were paying for it out of his or her own resources?
- If I am repeatedly troubled by a specific regulation or practice, have I sought ways to challenge the practice, substitute a more ethically acceptable practice, or bring the issue up for discussion?

I am fortunate to have been able to participate in the Woodstock Seminar and to explore with a group of enlightened and concerned individuals the ethical problems posed by the increasing complexity of the healthcare field. I wish every healthcare executive a similar opportunity, be it on a national, state, or local level.

Serving and Competing Ethically

Paul B. Hofmann, Dr.P.H., FACHE

REGARDLESS OF WHETHER a provider is not-for-profit or investor-owned, it has a formal mission statement and may have formal vision and value statements. However, if these documents fail to actually guide organizational and individual decision making, they are more than empty and meaningless rhetoric, they are symptoms of professional hypocrisy.

At a time when there is growing awareness that community and population-based health planning hold the best promise for improving community health status, many organizations are revisiting their mission statements.

At the same time, the growing influence of managed care, particularly capitation, has fostered sometimes fierce competition among providers. Even in those geographic areas where managed care has a relatively small penetration, excess bed capacity related to shorter lengths of stay and more outpatient surgery has stimulated aggressive marketing and advertising programs.

Serving and competing ethically in this environment is not impossible, but the challenge should not be underestimated. Promoting the best interest of the organization and serving the public's best interest are not always compatible objectives. For example, although unlikely in most situations, it is conceivable that a community's need might be best served if a hospital were to close. Similarly, an exceptionally successful marketing campaign that generates a significant increase in admission to one hospital could do so at the cost of irreparably compromising a competing hospital's ability to meet the needs of a largely medically indigent population.

Effective, ethical leaders are those who can sustain a delicate balance; they are able to achieve financial targets while maximizing community benefit. To help your healthcare organization meet its commitment to serve and compete ethically:

- Take measures to ensure that your mission, vision, and values statements are understood by every staff member and that decisions and actions are consistent with these statements.
- Ask yourself what the potential negative effects on the community will be and how they can be mitigated before embarking on competitive strategies.
- Avoid the temptation to excuse inefficient business practices by rationalizing that a not-for-profit organization need not adopt progressive and perhaps even aggressive policies and procedures.
- Actively engage board, management, and physician participation in any significant changes affecting the organization's image or role in the community.
- Evaluate the possible noneconomic as well as economic ramifications of reducing or eliminating programs or services.

Competition in healthcare is not inherently bad. Ultimately, we must remember that competition, like any other concept, can be distorted or abused. The fundamental ethical imperative for healthcare executives, regardless of institutional ownership, is to optimize the benefits of competition for the community as well as the organization.

The Ethics of Downsizing

Paul B. Hofmann, Dr.P.H., FACHE

Your organization has taken every possible step to become more cost-effective, but expenses must be reduced further, and it has become clear a significant number of positions will have to be eliminated. You have been designated as the management person responsible for designing the downsizing plan. How can your plan demonstrate genuine sensitivity to the ethical dimensions of this often painful process?

WHEN ADDRESSING THIS question, healthcare executives should first ask themselves, "What are my organization's objectives for downsizing and how can I measure my success in meeting them?"

Too often, a layoff plan has as its sole objective a reduction in workforce within a designated time frame to decrease salary and benefit costs. Frequently, department heads are requested to submit their proposals for meeting the designated figure, and the human resource director is held accountable for working with other senior executives to ensure appropriate coordination and implementation of these proposals after final approval by the CEO.

While it is important to determine specific downsizing targets, it is also necessary to develop additional objectives for the action.

Following are five you might consider adopting as well as appropriate measurement tools:

1. No diminution in quality of patient care. Measurement tool: results of patient satisfaction questionnaires, number and type of incident reports, patient complaints, and changes in other quality indicators.
2. A sustained level of productivity. Measurement tool: performance, absenteeism, and sick leave reports.
3. Retention of a positive image via focused communication efforts and other programs designed for patients, medical staff, board members, volunteers, and the community. Measurement tool: number of complaints, tone of media coverage, and other feedback.
4. Effective communication to and support for remaining and departing personnel. Measurement tool: post-layoff survey of current and former employees.
5. A reasonable severance package including appropriate length of severance payment and continuation of individual benefits (e.g., life insurance, disability insurance, medical benefits); provision of outplacement services; retraining support; and assistance with financial and/or retirement planning. Measurement tool: number of complaints, formal grievances, and wrongful discharge claims.

In a downsizing effort, management must not be morally neutral. Perhaps the most practical advice I can give is to capitalize on the past experiences of organizations that have dealt with this challenge. A particularly impressive report is "Hospital Layoffs: One Facility's Experience With a Work Force Reduction," by John D. Rudnick, Jr. (1995).

Also, to mitigate the anxiety and distress associated with downsizing measures, healthcare executives can employ a variety of formal actions that are described in ACHE's Ethical Policy Statement, "Ethical Issues Related to a Reduction in Force" [see Appendix B6]. Because almost every healthcare organization will have to reduce payroll costs, if it has not already done so, executives should review this policy statement carefully.

Employees deserve to be treated with fairness and integrity; therefore, executives should not use euphemisms to create insupportable illusions that everyone's needs will be met. Executives may want to refer to "restructuring" and "rightsizing," but these terms are transparent and ominous to the average employee. Feelings of apprehension, fear, and anger usually cannot be entirely eliminated; however, they can be at least partially alleviated by timely, consistent, and honest communication.

Recognizing
Conflicts of Interest

Laurence J. O'Connell Ph.D., S.T.D.

In the near future we will be sending out requests for proposals to bid on providing mental health services to members of our managed care network. I am friends with the CEO of one of the acknowledged best providers of this service in our area. From a management perspective, I believe the provider should be included in the bidding process, but I am concerned this move might be perceived as a conflict of interest. How can I best fulfill my management and ethical responsibility in this case?

THIS QUESTION HIGHLIGHTS two important issues that should be front and center in the ethical analysis of any business transaction. First, the distinction between perceived and actual wrongdoing must be carefully evaluated. Second, the respective demands of personal integrity and professional responsibility should be acknowledged, respected, and sensitively resolved. The interplay of perception, personal morality, and professional obligation is frequently the source of ethical ambiguity in the workplace. It is thus essential to sort out their moral frontiers as they present themselves in a particular situation and to balance the legitimate and ethically compelling claims of each.

In this case, the most basic requirement of personal morality has already been met; the executive's own moral sensitivity and insight brought the issues to light. The point is quite simple: Moral consciousness is more or less developed in each of us. Our ability to recognize and actively deal with the moral dimensions of any situation depends on the level of moral development we have achieved. Developing our moral reasoning is a life-long project that ideally leads to increasing degrees of practical wisdom. It does not just happen. It requires effort and a fundamental disposition to do what is right and good.

Since healthcare executives often wield immense power that affects the well-being of individuals and society, sensitive moral reasoning should be listed among their indispensable competencies. Yet, good moral sense is just the foundation of ethical behavior. It will not make decision making any easier or professional life any less complicated.

The relationship between the executive and the CEO of the mental health provider is a good example of such complications. It alerts us to a potential conflict that pits one set of legitimate interests against another, and it invites us to search for ethically important factors. For example, the nature of the relationship may be morally relevant. If the executive is romantically involved with the CEO of the mental health provider or owns an equity position in his company, the strong potential for a genuine conflict of interest exists.

Nevertheless, the executive has a fiduciary responsibility to ensure the quality of mental health services in her managed care network. Standard professional ethics demand that she find the best service with the resources made available. This obligation would require gathering bids from the broadest range of potential providers. Thus, even if there were a perception of favoritism should she choose her friend's company, she is still obliged to consider his bid. To dismiss his bid out of hand because it might be perceived as wrongdoing could violate her fiduciary duty to her own organization and impose an unjust restraint upon her friend's company. Here we have the makings of a genuine moral dilemma that graphically displays the sometimes shadowy mix of public perceptions, personal morality, and professional ethics.

In this case, the company should formulate, approve, and publicize a process and criteria for selecting providers. It could also establish a blind process, considering all bids on their merits, apart from knowledge of the companies' names. To the extent that company records are needed to establish merit or to meet other selection criteria, a modified blind process may be required. In this situation, one or more individuals would have the responsibility of reviewing and summarizing the required information.

In another approach, the concerned executive could remove herself from both the review and selection process, thereby avoiding what some might otherwise perceive to be a conflict of interest, collusion, or rigged bidding. If this service provider really is one of the best, comes in with a competitive bid, and is selected, the executive should frankly—and without moral qualms—support the choice by appeals to the best interests of her network members and the integrity of her selection process.

The rapid pace and organizational complexity of today's healthcare environment inevitably spawns these ambiguous situations in which personal and professional interests intersect in often unexpected and sometimes explosive ways. Moral quandaries are part of today's professional landscape. While they are unavoidable, they are neither intractable nor as threatening as they first appear.

A few broader notions can guide thinking. Personal integrity should be bolstered by organizational integrity. Corporate policies and procedures should be designed to promote responsible decision making in morally charged situations in which several legitimate interests are at stake. Moreover, corporate leaders with a strong sense of personal integrity can be moral exemplars. It should be possible to communicate the reasoned, explicit, and conscious values that they use to support choices, commitments, and styles. In this way, one life lived with integrity will filter to others and gradually seep into the essence of corporate culture. Personal integrity and wise business choices need not oppose one another.

Beyond the Margin

Michael G. Daigneault, Esq.

As the CEO of a not-for-profit healthcare system, I am struggling to find a balance between my responsibility to my organization and to my community. Obviously, my system is expected to operate in the black; it also, however, is committed to providing care to the poor and underserved. How do I balance these two seemingly contradictory responsibilities?

OFTEN, IN THE examples used to teach ethical decision making, the inherent conflicts in the ethical dilemmas are relatively simple. For example, value conflicts are often demonstrated with hypothetical questions such as: Is it acceptable to steal a loaf of bread to feed a starving child? Is it okay to tell someone that she "looks wonderful" when her age or illness is making her look less than terrific? In these cases, the dilemma is quite clear.

In the case stated here, there *appears* to be a dilemma: fiscal responsibility versus community service. However, the underlying question is whether these "seemingly contradictory responsibilities" are, in fact, in conflict.

The issue is that healthcare systems must foster their overall financial well-being while maintaining certain services to the community that do not in themselves produce a positive revenue stream. Segments of healthcare such as emergency services, neonatal care, mental health services, and, yes, care for the poor are not particularly cost-effective. Though there is sometimes little or no margin for these particular services, it does not mean they should be eliminated.

At the same time, operating "in the black" is an essential obligation of any healthcare organization. As the Sisters of Mercy are frequently noted as saying, "no margin, no mercy." This does not mean that margin is, or should be, the *raison d'être* of a healthcare organization. It does suggest, however, that "margin" is a necessary, but insufficient, precondition to success. It is the raw material of caring for the poor and underserved.

As with any of the community's other competing needs, the economic burden that any healthcare system must bear to help the underserved must be fairly and appropriately balanced and managed. But it is a burden that should and must be borne.

Why? Because the bond of trust that exists between healthcare providers and the communities they serve goes far beyond mandated legal or business obligations—individuals have no other viable choice but to depend on the existing healthcare system in their community. Because of that special trust, healthcare providers must conduct all their medical and business activities in a caring and ethical manner.

This argues for the proposition that all healthcare organizations bear a collective responsibility to meet the healthcare needs of the communities they serve. There will likely always be a dynamic tension between the needs of a community and the capacity of any healthcare organization, hospital, or healthcare system to meet those needs. But this does not preclude a healthcare organization from meeting its own business and financial objectives.

In other words, there may not be an ethical dilemma here, at least not at the macro level. At the highest level, these values—financial responsibility and community service—are not in conflict; rather, one is a precondition needed to support the other.

There is often tension between these values, however, as there never seems to be enough money to do all that we could or would do to serve society. Every organization has at one time maintained that it could do more if only it had more time, people, and money.

At the macro level, we know that not everyone can get everything they want every time they want it. But that is little solace as we agonize over whether to commit resources to meet a given individual's needs. The best we can strive to accomplish, as we balance both margin and mercy, is to allocate our limited resources in ways that optimize the value we give to society—that do the most good for the greatest number.

In practical terms, doing so may, in some cases, limit our services to the necessities of saving lives and easing pain. We may desire to do more to add quality to the lives of those we serve, not just longevity. We may wish to save the leg, not just the life. We may wish to heal the wound and leave no scar. But we do not get all that we wish for. We cannot save the leg if doing so costs another's life. It is the fundamental lesson of triage: finite resources spread over a great need.

We may despair and wish it were not so, but it is. How do we balance what at first glance appear to be contradictory responsibilities? As best we can—with humanity and humility. But balance them we must. If we fail to provide for either margin or mercy today, we will fail to provide for both of them tomorrow.

Downsizing:
Confidentiality vs. Disclosure

Paul B. Hofmann, Dr.P.H., FACHE

I am a senior manager at a mid-sized healthcare organization. My vice president told me recently that, as part of a restructuring effort, our organization will be laying off a significant number of staff. Rumors of the downsizing have gotten out, and a few managers and other staff who report to me have asked me if the rumors are true. I know I have a responsibility to keep management's confidence, but what about my responsibility to my employees who will soon be out of work?

FIRST, IT IS important to consider why the vice president would want to keep the downsizing decision confidential. The reasons probably include: the expectation that morale will plummet; the fear that some of the most valued employees will take positions elsewhere; the concern that productivity will decline and patient care will be affected; the possibility that the media will publicize the decision and raise difficult questions; or the need for more time to develop a comprehensive layoff policy, determine appropriate severance benefits and outplacement procedures, and prepare a detailed communications plan. (Although, as emphasized in ACHE's Ethical Policy Statement, "Ethical Issues Related to a Reduction in Force," organizations should develop formal policies and procedures on downsizing "well in advance of the need to implement them.")

These reasons are valid, but their legitimacy would not justify denying that downsizing will occur when you know such a decision has been made. That would not only be dishonest from a personal standpoint, but would also compromise your credibility and employees' trust in management overall. When the truth emerges, management will have discouraged employee initiative and creativity at a time when they are most needed.

Your employees have a right to receive accurate, timely, clear, and consistent information about developments affecting their job status. In his book *Reorganization and Renewal: Strategies for Healthcare Leaders,* Donald N. Lombardi, Ph.D. (1997), dedicates a chapter to downsizing. He describes the need for decency, accuracy, forthrightness, compassion, fortitude, introspection, and commitment, and describes why they are so relevant in downsizing. In addition, he discusses the classic reactions employees exhibit when downsizing is announced: anger, victimization, passivity, shock, resentfulness, fear, vengeance, embarrassment, and betrayal.

It is simply unrealistic to assume that most if not all of these feelings are avoidable. Therefore, failure to anticipate and address them will only exacerbate their associated consequences.

So how should this particular situation be handled? You might respond, "I have heard the same rumors and will ask the executive staff to address them as quickly as possible." With this reply, you have kept management's confidence, have not been dishonest to your subordinates, and yet have promised to take immediate action. Once you have made that promise, you must follow up on it: As soon as you are able, communicate the details of the downsizing to your staff, and be prepared to deal with the reactions that follow.

The Ethics of Diversity

John Abbott Worthley, D.P.A.

A team from my organization is planning a meeting with a potential client. Because this client strongly values diversity, we want our team to represent the diversity of our organization. I am considering inviting a number of young executives to participate; however, some of them are being included on the team primarily because of their minority status. This meeting could be a valuable experience for all who participate, but I am concerned about including individuals on the basis of their race or sex. What are my ethical responsibilities to these employees and to the organization?

THE SITUATION YOU describe has several significant dimensions. Clearly, there are political, legal, organizational, and financial elements. Politically, cultural diversity and affirmative action are headline issues. This situation is the sort of thing that can get an organization in the news if mishandled. Legally, recent court cases have highlighted problems of reverse discrimination stemming from affirmative action efforts. Lawsuits are now not unlikely when situations like this are managed injudiciously. Organizationally, "career-enhancing" opportunities such as this can tend to focus attention on race or sex rather than ability, often leading to

175

resentment among staff. On the other hand, your organization stands to benefit financially from making a good impression on this potential client. The political, legal, organizational, and financial elements stand out and can easily block out other considerations. But there is another dimension to this situation—the ethical dimension—and it may well overarch the others.

In probing the ethical dimension of an issue, you might first identify and clarify the values at stake. For example, one of the values that should be considered in this situation is your organization's well-being; the organization has a significant interest in pleasing the potential client. On the other hand, fairness to all—including avoidance of discrimination—also needs to be honored. The political, legal, and organizational dimensions of this situation are all related to the value of fairness. Also at stake are the values of honesty and competence, which need to be honored in the ethical dimension. It is one thing to honestly represent an organization's diversity; it is another thing to misrepresent it. Inviting young executives who are competent is one thing; inviting some who are not is another matter.

In this situation, as in all ethically charged situations, it is your ethical responsibility to honor all of these values, although some may seem to be in competition. For example, honoring the organization's well-being requires attention to the diversity issues in dealing with this client; but honoring the dignity of these young executives may require inclusion based only on professional competence, not on race or sex. Meeting your ethical responsibility requires a search for options, one of which might reconcile otherwise competing values. Discussing the situation with the people involved is an option that usually helps to clarify the issue.

Addressing your ethical responsibility is certainly much more difficult in the short term than simply going all out for the organization's interest, or backing off from fear of employee, community, or legal reaction. In the long run, however, pursuit of your ethical responsibilities may well be the key to effectively managing the political, legal, organizational, and financial dimensions. As we are hearing more and more in the corporate world, good ethics may, indeed, be good business.

Work vs. Family

Lawrence B. Chonko, Ph.D.

I recently interviewed for department head positions at two different organizations, one nearby and one in another state. The out-of-state organization offered me a position, and I accepted it verbally. A few days later, the in-state organization offered me a position as well. This one pays a bit more, and my family would not have to move. I know I have an obligation to keep my word to the first organization, but I also have an obligation to my spouse and children. How can I make this decision in an ethical manner?

THIS SITUATION INVOLVES three primary ethics—your individual ethic, a professional ethic, and an organizational ethic. Your individual ethic plays a part in the way such values as integrity, equality of opportunity, and freedom to make our own decisions will impact the final outcome of any ethical decision situation. At the same time, the professional ethic emphasizes the norms of the profession; in essence, the professional ethic asks the question, "What would most of my colleagues do?" Finally, the organizational ethic addresses the goals of an organization and whether an individual is acting in the organization's best interests. Additionally, in this case, your family considerations may act as a fourth ethic—probably the most difficult aspect of this decision.

Consider this dilemma with the first three ethics in mind. First, as a person of integrity, the individual ethic of this decision would dictate that your word be your bond. Second, under the professional ethic, or the norms of your profession, a verbal acceptance is a type of contract—to renege might not be illegal, but it would certainly be unethical and unprofessional. Finally, retracting your acceptance would also violate the organizational ethic, as it would not be in the organization's best interests.

For these reasons, your ethical obligation, at this point, is to stop searching and turn down any future interview requests and job offers after accepting any new job. Your decision should be final. Make sure that you stand by it.

Of course, this is not to disregard the needs of your family. Those considerations, however, should have been included at all levels of this career decision, from initial contact with the employer to your acceptance of the offer. By considering the family issues early on, difficult choices such as this would be eased. In the future, the following advice can help you minimize the conflict associated with similar ethical decisions:

Don't put yourself in a difficult situation. Know what you are looking for from each prospective employer. Know what trade-offs you are willing to make, and before accepting any offer, evaluate the organization based on your criteria and your tolerance limits.

Beware of selective perception. We sometimes tend to consider only those factors that support the choice we want to make and ignore those that would steer us toward another option. Be sure to consider all the factors that could influence your decision.

Plan your time well. A deadline on a decision may bias your judgment and limit the amount of information you take in. Work out a schedule with all affected parties so that you have enough time to make an educated decision.

In this situation, some advance thinking about your needs, time constraints, and family considerations may have prevented this dilemma. This is why it is important to judiciously and painstakingly consider your own needs as well as those of your family and the organizations that will be influenced and are influential in your decision.

Allocating Limited Capital Resources

Paul B. Hofmann, Dr.P.H., FACHE

Predictably, we always receive more project requests than can be accommodated by our capital budget. In addition to the traditional financial criteria, are there ethical factors that should be considered when a choice must be made among equally compelling requests?

INVARIABLY, HEALTHCARE EXECUTIVES are asked to approve capital expenditures in excess of available funds. And given the unrelenting economic pressures to provide more services with less reimbursement, this situation will not abate in the near future.

CONVENTIONAL APPROACH

Historically, decision makers have relied almost exclusively on well-tested criteria to assess the impact of a proposed project or piece of equipment, including:

- Meeting the needs of various constituencies (patients, physicians, employees, and others)
- Improving the cost-effectiveness of service (including safety, length of stay, access, and productivity)

- Complying with legal, licensing, regulatory, and Joint Commission requirements
- Satisfying financial viability measures (time period to obtain return on investment, contribution margin per case, probability of achieving forecast)

The use of these and similar evaluation criteria to make an objective, sound decision is both appropriate and essential, but not sufficient. This is especially true when you are confronted with proposals that appear equally compelling. A comprehensive cost-benefit comparison should be complemented by an ethical analysis. The ultimate goal, of course, is to make decisions that are not only economically justified but also morally defensible.

APPLICATION OF ETHICAL PRINCIPLES

A review of the literature on ethics and ethical theory suggests that a wide range of ethical principles could be relevant to the capital budget decision-making process; however, the following four have specific relevance.

1. *Beneficence* could be defined as acting with charity and kindness, but this definition is inadequate. Fully embracing the principle requires actively promoting behaviors that benefit others. The key term here is "active"; passivity fundamentally violates the basic integrity of the concept. With many nonprofit hospitals vulnerable to allegations that they do not provide sufficient community benefit to justify their tax-exempt status, the ability of some organizations to literally document their beneficence may influence long-term organizational survival.
2. *Nonmaleficence* prohibits doing harm to others. A healthcare executive has an indisputable obligation to take no action that would injure the organization or those it serves. For example, by

avoiding misconduct that could result in compromising the organization and its staff, management refuses to engage in activities that might represent a conflict of interest. This is not simply a hypothetical concern. Capital expenditure decisions could easily be made that may have personal and/or institutional value to the detriment of the community, such as supporting a project advocated by a board member rather than funding an indigent care clinic.

3. *Fidelity* suggests adherence to a contract or covenant to fulfill certain responsibilities. This principle also connotes fulfilling one's duty and keeping promises. In the context of deciding among competing proposals, all of them being highly desirable, which one will be most supportive of the organization's overall mission and values? A thoughtful, dispassionate examination of each proposal's relevance to sustaining the current and future mission should be an indispensable part of the analysis. Similarly, if a request is not aligned with your organization's values, it should compare unfavorably with competing applications for capital funds.

4. *Justice* implies a responsibility to act with fairness and impartiality. Although it is difficult to argue that any of the principles should "trump" another, an appropriate resource allocation decision cannot be made unless it is fair and impartial. Not only should the distribution of resources reflect fairness, but the outcome should also consider the legacy of previous inequities. Consequently, justice mandates a complete exploration of the moral traces resulting from past practices of discrimination, as well as activities that were influenced by different circumstances and priorities. Earlier appropriation decisions could have been affected by political factors that are no longer applicable. These past actions must be taken into consideration when making resource allocation decisions today.

Healthcare executives, like those in other fields, practice the fine art of the possible, becoming ever more proficient in making organizational compromises by negotiating politically acceptable solutions. Determining which capital proposals will be approved when all cannot be funded, regardless of their sound justification, often requires a delicate balancing process. The more thorough and comprehensive the assessment, incorporating both economic and noneconomic criteria, the more likely the outcome will be both prudent and just.

PART IX

Institutional Resources

Creating an Effective Ethics Program

David L. Perry

WHAT STEPS CAN healthcare executives take to develop and implement a comprehensive, long-term initiative in organizational ethics? Here are the measures recommended by the Ethics Resource Center, a private, not-for-profit corporation based in Washington, DC.

Assess organizational values and vulnerabilities to misconduct. Many organizations make the mistake of assigning a small group of staff (usually from the legal department) to write a code of ethics without first making any attempt to find out what kinds of ethical issues employees *really* face in their day-to-day jobs. Not only does an inadequate up-front organizational assessment result in a weak and irrelevant code of ethics, it also means that management remains ignorant of the kinds of problems that can't be addressed in a code alone.

Management simply can't afford not to know, for example, whether the organization's goal-setting practices, incentive and reward systems, and performance evaluations encourage *ethical* conduct or *undermine* it. It does little good to state in a code of ethics that quality and safety are paramount if in practice employees are consistently rewarded only for cutting costs. Making the effort to identify employee *values* can provide the foundation for consensus on the organization's fundamental ethical principles.

Create opportunities for management to discuss organizational values and risks. Data emerging from an organizational assessment will often call for developing clear standards of conduct, employee training, and changing management systems and practices, etc. Management must reach consensus on the high-priority issues as well as action plans that must be formulated to tackle those issues head-on. If management does not develop a strong sense of ownership of the ethics program, employees will perceive it to be merely a temporary fad and not a long-term commitment.

Develop and communicate clear standards of conduct. Once management understands the issues, a written code of ethics can be created or revised. This code should relate to management systems and practices. In addition, the code should affirm a basic set of organizational values, principles or commitments, establish ground rules in areas where they are needed, provide illustrations and guidelines in some of the "gray" areas, and explain how employees can obtain further advice and counsel without fear of retribution. New-employee orientations should include a healthy dose of instruction in the organization's ethical standards and ethics-related case studies. In addition, ongoing discussions should be woven into managerial training courses.

Refine management systems and practices to support the ethics program. This is at once the most difficult and the most important step because it gets at the basic tools that managers use to manage: goal-setting (strategic, departmental, individual); incentive and reward systems; performance appraisals; and disciplinary practices. All of these practices need to be evaluated according to whether they serve to reinforce the ethics program. This isn't a single step, but an ongoing process of refinement and improvement.

Ethics development is not just attending a training program or reading the code of conduct. Ethics has to do with the organization's basic culture and operating values—the pride and satisfaction employees find in their work, the attention to quality and service, the degree to which suppliers and customers are treated fairly and honestly—all of which impinge upon the organization's overall reputation and success.

Performing an Ethics Audit

Paul B. Hofmann, Dr.P.H., FACHE

WHILE FINANCIAL AUDITS have been commonplace for decades, a comparable process for examining documents and activity in the context of ethical implications is not common in healthcare or in other fields. Enter the ethics audit—a formal process of reviewing an organization's policies, procedures, and outcomes from an ethical perspective. The ethics audit is an effective way to ensure that your organization is fulfilling its mission, even in the most demanding times.

WARNING SIGNS

The best time to conduct an ethics audit is when no apparent crisis exists. Indeed, one of the principal objectives of performing an audit is to identify potential difficulties and to address them before they become serious problems. When does an ethics audit become critical? Although no single issue or problem serves as a key indicator, an organization should seriously consider an ethics audit if there is even a small increase in:

- employee grievances, resignations, terminations, and wrongful discharge complaints;
- patient complaints, incident reports, and legal actions;
- medical staff complaints and resignations;
- problems with suppliers and other vendors; or
- adverse publicity.

CONDUCTING AN AUDIT

The first step in conducting an ethics audit is the collection and analysis of key documents. These documents include the organization's mission, vision, and values statements as well as the portions of its policy and procedures manual covering issues such as uncompensated care, confidentiality, conflicts of interest, and sexual harassment.

The next step requires surveying representative board members, management staff, physicians, employees, volunteers, and community residents and organizations. Conducted through a structured questionnaire, the surveys should reinforce the organization's commitment to ethical behavior and at the same time determine where there have been inconsistencies between formal policy statements and perceived or actual performance.

The third step is to develop and implement educational programs that address apparent problems. For example, if your mission statement supports working with your community but survey results indicate a perception that your organization is working in isolation, you can take the appropriate steps to educate stakeholders about the organization's efforts to promote community involvement.

If you determine that the problem is more than a communication issue, you can begin to develop specific strategies to enhance community involvement.

As another means of eliminating ethical inconsistencies, health-care organizations can create and disseminate an ethics manual. For instance, 3M has prepared a business conduct manual to reemphasize its corporate values and assist the company in "maintaining the highest ethical standards in all its business operations." In addition, 3M has established a toll-free Business Conduct Information Line to address employee questions regarding company policies and receive incident reports. Finally, ACHE's *Code of Ethics* is an ideal guide for ethical conduct in healthcare management.

For organizations seeking additional resources on ethics and healthcare management, I highly recommend *Ethical Considerations in the Business Aspects of Health Care* (Woodstock Theological Center 1995).

Appointing an Ethics Officer

Edward Petry, Ph.D.

As my organization grows increasingly complex, so do the ethical dilemmas we face. Would appointing an ethics officer help us clarify these issues? What responsibilities would be inherent to this position?

IN RESPONSE TO heightened government scrutiny, increasing application of the False Claims Act, and widespread publicity given to scandals and investigations, many healthcare organizations today are asking these questions. Increasingly, they are concluding that they need to review their internal ethics initiatives and appoint an executive to manage these programs.

Responsibilities of an ethics officer generally include managing internal reporting systems, assessing ethics risk areas, developing and distributing ethics policies and publications, investigating alleged violations, and designing training programs. Because ethics and compliance programs have similar foundations, in some organizations the ethics officer might manage compliance functions as well.

Because these responsibilities are far-reaching, this position should be primarily a management one and not just a policing and/or legal function. While ethics officers are often highly placed in the organization, the officer and the ethics program must also be backed up by other senior managers.

Smaller, single-facility healthcare organizations may be able to manage their ethics programs as a function of the human resources division. However, given the complexity of ethical dilemmas encountered in today's healthcare environment and the seriousness of the consequences if violations do occur, large, multi-site systems would be well-served by appointing an ethics officer.

If your organization chooses to do so, be aware that partial measures are not enough. Too often, a large, complex organization believes that by appointing a part-time, mid-level ethics officer, it will be able to address any ethical concerns that develop. Increasingly, however, such efforts are being viewed with suspicion. In a survey of Ethics Officer Association members, who represent more than 30 u.s. industries, part-time ethics officers reported an average of 96 annual contacts, including questions about policies as well as allegations of wrongdoing; full-time ethics officers, however, reported an average of 1,486 annual contacts. Some of this disparity might exist because employees believe part-time programs indicate a lack of organizational commitment to ethics. More wholehearted efforts, however, can help communicate an organization's dedication to ethical practices. In fact, a study by Walker Information found that when organizations provide ethics information resources such as a code of ethics, a value statement, and/or an ethics officer, employees rate them as highly ethical.

Today, every organization needs to examine its level of commitment to internal ethics by asking the following:

- Are we keeping up with the ethical standards of our field?
- Do we have a plan to keep pace with the rising expectations of the public, employees, and regulators?
- Are we providing adequate resources, guidance, and support to help our employees make difficult ethical decisions?

- Would an employee know where to turn in our organization to get help with an ethical dilemma?
- Would they be willing to report a possible violation without fear of retaliation?
- Are we taking all necessary steps to prevent and detect violation of law, regulations, and corporate policies?

If the answer to any of these questions is "no," consider learning from other organizations who have already been down this road.

Beyond Compliance

Liz Whitley, Ph.D., and Gerry Heeley, S.T.D

My organization is beginning to develop a compliance program. While such a program can ensure that the organization's activities are legal, I'm not sure that compliance alone is enough. Aren't there ethical obligations beyond compliance, and if so, how can we incorporate ethics into our compliance plan?

GIVEN THE RECENT emphasis on compliance—as well as the consequences of noncompliance—in healthcare management today, many healthcare executives understandably are fixated on this issue. However, while a compliance program may address some ethical issues, a healthcare organization's obligation to act ethically extends beyond a compliance program's reach. The best way to ensure that your organization is able to meet its legal and ethical standards is to create compliance and ethics programs that complement each other.

If a compliance program is to meet its goals of preventing, detecting, and addressing illegal conduct, it must include the development and distribution of written standards of compliance, the appointment of a compliance officer, training and education of employees, monitoring and enforcement, investigating misconduct, and procedures for corrective action. Properly implemented, a compliance program supports conformity to legal and regulatory requirements, and in the event of misconduct, may reduce penalties, according to the Federal Sentencing Guidelines.

However, the limitations of a compliance program are numerous. First, conduct that is legal may not necessarily be ethical. Additionally, the emphasis on punishment may have a negative effect on employee morale and trust in management. Preoccupation with externally imposed standards does not evoke excellence or guide exemplary behavior.

An ethics program can expand upon a compliance program. The two have some common features, but an ethics strategy must also include a companywide commitment to creating a culture that inspires ethical behavior and encourages integrity. This is not something that will happen on its own—it requires a significant commitment from management and involves all members of the organization.

Although concerned with legal and regulatory compliance, the primary goal of an ethics program should be to foster exemplary ethical behavior. Its benefits include self-governance according to chosen standards; improved communication, decision making, and cooperation throughout the organization; and enhanced reputation and relationships with the community.

To develop an ethics program that works in conjunction with your compliance plan, some strategies you might consider include:

- Adopting a continuous quality improvement approach to communicating and living your organization's mission and core values
- Training senior executives to incorporate ethical considerations into daily activities and interactions with staff
- Educating staff, through large-group presentations and small-group discussion, on the ethics and compliance plans

- Developing tools and techniques for including ethics as a criterion for hiring and promotion
- Including ethics on every meeting agenda throughout the organization

Integrating your compliance program with an ethics program, though not required, is highly recommended. Compliance programs endorse a universal legal and regulatory approach to behavior in healthcare organizations. Ethics programs, on the other hand, encourage exemplary behavior based on the unique culture or character of your organization.

Evaluating Your Ethics Committees

William A. Nelson, Ph.D.

THE IMPORTANCE, GOALS, and functions of healthcare ethics committees are clearly evolving in relation to the changing healthcare environment. Historically, ethics committees have been acute-care oriented, often confronting ethical medical dilemmas related to the end of life. Today, healthcare organizations are becoming increasingly primary care and outpatient focused—and the distinction between bedside and boardroom ethical issues is becoming increasingly blurred. In response, ethics committees are being required to widen their scope to include clinical and organizational ethics alike. In an era of managed care, ethics committees must be capable of addressing such issues as the allocation of hospital resources or the role of clinicians as gatekeepers. In other words, they must confront broader mission, policy, and procedural concerns, not just individual patient issues.

As the complexity and urgency of ethical healthcare issues escalate, your organization may increasingly turn to its ethics committee for guidance and direction. To determine if your ethics committee is positioned to act effectively, review the following dimensions of your committee.

All ethics committee members, as well as your organization's staff and administration, should understand and accept the purpose and functions of the committee. To evaluate how clearly the ethics committee's purpose is defined, ask committee members to answer this question: "What is the purpose of our committee?"

This question often elicits surprisingly different responses, even if the group has been working together for several years. Before gaining organizationwide support, you must achieve consensus within the committee as to its purpose and goals.

Once the committee's purpose is defined and accepted, establish clear guidelines regarding how the ethics committee performs its functions, including policy review, education, evaluation, and clinical/organizational ethics consultations. For example, how will the committee carry out its ethics consultations? Does the whole committee consult on an issue, or does a smaller team respond? Who on the committee does staff contact with ethical concerns? To determine how informed your staff is about your ethics committee, ask individuals in various departments how they would access the ethics committee and what they would expect to accomplish by consulting it. You may discover that you need to educate staff about the ethics committee's purpose and processes so that its potential as an internal resource is maximized. Without clarity and acceptance of purpose, functions, and structure, your ethics committee may not be perceived as a useful resource.

COMPOSITION AND COMPETENCIES OF MEMBERS

Broad and balanced professional representation is essential for your committee to be respected and used by your staff and administration. Because cultural perspective influences how people approach illness, ethics committee membership should reflect the diversity of the healthcare organization and the community it serves. For example, if a dominant religious or ethnic population is being served by your organization, those communities must be represented by the ethics committee membership. Furthermore, to ensure active participation by its members, ethics committees should be composed primarily of volunteers, rather than individuals who are assigned to serve on the committee. Recruit new members by identifying individuals in your organization who show interest and demonstrate reasoned thinking regarding ethical issues. Survey staff and coworkers, and take note of those who participate in common educational activities that pertain to ethical issues.

In addition to possessing interest, motivation, and time, the best ethics committee members will be those who possess a comprehensive set of competencies. The American Society for Bioethics and Humanities' (1998) report, "Core Competencies for Health Care Ethics Consultation," offers guidelines for the appropriate knowledge, skills, and character for those performing ethics consultations. The report identifies three major skill sets:

1. *Ethical assessment skills* enable individuals to identify the values underlying ethical conflicts. These skills include the ability to distinguish the ethical dimensions of a situation from other overlapping dimensions, such as legal or medical; to access, critically evaluate, and use relevant knowledge; to identify and justify various morally acceptable options and their consequences; and to evaluate evidence and arguments for and against different solutions.
2. *Process skills* focus on efforts to resolve the uncertainty related to values that arises in healthcare settings. These skills include the ability to facilitate meetings, identify key decision makers, create an atmosphere of trust, negotiate between competing moral views, and engage in creative problem solving.

3. *Interpersonal skills* include the ability to listen effectively, educate concerned parties about the ethical dimensions of their dilemma, and represent the views of concerned parties to others.

In addition to these general skills, the report identified nine core knowledge areas that are required for competent ethical consultation. Your ethics committee should be populated by individuals who possess some level of knowledge in these areas, which include an understanding of the following:

1. Moral reasoning and ethical theory
2. Common bioethical issues and concepts
3. Healthcare systems, including knowledge of managed care and governmental systems
4. Clinical context
5. Your healthcare organization, including the organization's mission statement and structure
6. Your healthcare organization's policies
7. Beliefs and perspectives of the local patient and staff population
8. Relevant codes of ethics and professional conduct and guidelines of accrediting organizations
9. Relevant health law

In addition to this knowledge, ethics consultants—similar to all healthcare professionals—should possess and exhibit good character such as tolerance, honesty, courage, prudence, and integrity.

LEADERSHIP

The chairperson of your ethics committee must be well respected within your organization, have a comprehensive understanding of the organization's formal and informal decision-making processes and be open to input and feedback from committee members and staff. To keep your ethics committee viable and dynamic, the chairperson should not be a "fixture"; in other words, he or she should not hold the position to the point where the committee becomes dependent on that individual. The committee should be structured so that all members actively contribute and tasks are fairly distributed.

ORGANIZATIONAL SUPPORT AND RESPECT

To ensure quality in the functions of the ethics committee, your organization must support and respect its role. Administration and trustees should help ethics committee members develop competencies by providing educational resources and ensuring that members are given adequate time for their ethics committee duties. Furthermore, it is crucial that the organization create a climate for the committee to carry out its activities with integrity. The committee should not be expected to simply echo the organization's position on certain issues; rather, they must be able to speak freely in an appropriate and tactful manner, regardless of the organization's stance. Only then will honest dialogue take place between the administration and the committee to enhance the overall ethical nature of the organization.

Ethics committees that are well informed, representative, and motivated can be a healthcare organization's greatest resource for ethical guidance and support.

The Ethics of Compliance Hotlines

John Abbott Worthley, D.P.A.

My organization's compliance program has built-in mechanisms that include an anonymous "hotline" for informing management of suspected misconduct as well as more direct written and verbal channels. Our compliance officer and senior management stress the importance of using these vehicles, but I am concerned that overuse could put innocent people in embarrassing situations. What is my ethical responsibility regarding the extent to which I should encourage my staff to use these mechanisms?

THIS QUESTION PROVOCATIVELY illustrates the way compliance ethics can intersect with organizational ethics. To uphold compliance responsibilities, healthcare organizations need effective ways to prevent, detect, and address violations of laws, regulations, and standards. Anonymous hotlines are common compliance mechanisms, and the knowledge that such hotlines exist tends to discourage noncompliant behavior. When the hotlines are used, they can detect noncompliant actions—information healthcare organizations can use to address problems. Consequently, it is likely that your compliance officer and senior executives stress the importance of informant mechanisms such as a hotline.

As you suggest with your question, however, compliance realities and responsibilities often go hand-in-hand with organizational ethics realities and responsibilities. While the former tend to focus on legality and honesty, organizational ethics are broader. They hold that fairness and human dignity need vigilant attention. That is why you—as indicated in your question—are trying to highlight these latter values. The tension you are experiencing is the classic conflict between the common good (in this case, organizational well-being) and individual rights (fairness and dignity). Balancing these values is one of the greatest challenges facing healthcare executives today, and succeeding requires managerial creativity and practical measures. Your ethical responsibility, in a nutshell, is to provide the operational means for protecting all these important values.

How can we build into hotlines processes that will prevent, detect, and address misuse of the informant mechanism? By misuse, of course, I mean precisely what your question concerns: unfairly subjecting innocent employees to embarrassing situations. Responding to this challenge calls for creative thinking. Some possibilities include the following:

- *Due process procedures:* Our legal system's concern for fairness and dignity has led to rigorous requirements of notice, hearing, and appeal for anyone charged with a crime. Creatively adapting these time-honored due process principles to organizational compliance systems is one avenue for you to explore. For example, you can give alleged offenders formal hearings before action is taken against them, as well as implement a formal appeals process if an action is decided.
- *Nomenclature:* Some companies have addressed this challenge by avoiding the term "hotline." Instead, names such as "helpline" or "guideline" have been used; these suggest a dialogue of advice and counsel in which unwarranted reports

might be screened while nonthreatening anonymity is maintained.

- *Confidentiality:* Studies have shown that for reporting mechanisms to be effective, nonretaliatory assurances are essential. Thus, confidentiality through anonymity for the informer is critical. The same sort of rigorous confidentiality can be given to the person accused. One way to preserve anonymity is hire an outside firm to manage the hotline.

- *Training:* An important way to meet the challenge is to institute rigorous ethics training in your department. This training should reflect equally on the importance of legality and fairness, and sensitize employees to the importance of both reporting suspected violations and avoiding frivolous accusations.

In the end, this matter will be an ongoing managerial issue because of the conflicting interests involved. Too much emphasis on avoiding unwarranted accusations can weaken a hotline's effectiveness; permitting too much carefree use can lead to abuse. Your ethical responsibility is to stress both with equal rigor by providing mechanisms that facilitate openness and fairness.

Improving Ethics Committee Effectiveness

Paul B. Hofmann, Dr.P.H., FACHE

We have a well-organized ethics committee that has produced useful policies, consulted on cases, and sponsored education programs for both the staff and the community. Nonetheless, case consultation requests are rare, and we feel that the committee's resources in other areas are not used to their potential. What should we do?

YOUR CONCERNS ARE not uncommon. Many ethics committees are struggling with their role, confused about their responsibilities beyond the traditional focus on clinical issues. The rising interest in organizational, business, and management ethics, along with corporate compliance, has prompted ethics committees to reassess their goals and objectives.

When hospital executives were asked at an ACHE seminar (in 2000) if the ethics committees in their organizations were highly effective, very few individuals replied affirmatively. Consequently, it is not surprising that committee members may be questioning their value to the organization.

Your staff may not be making the most of your ethics committee for a variety of reasons. Among them are:

- Inaccurate understanding of the committee's role and potential contribution. Some staff members may think the committee's sole function is to provide case consultation when there is concern about an end-of-life dilemma. Others may hesitate to ask for assistance because they do not want to be obligated to comply with the ethics committee's conclusion, failing to realize that the committee is an advisory, not a decision-making, body. Still others may be concerned about conveying extremely sensitive information, not recognizing the committee's efforts to preserve nondisclosure and confidentiality.
- Low visibility. Depending on the location of your committee in your organizational structure, publicity about its purpose, and periodic reports on its activity, many people may be unaware of its existence and the resource it represents.
- Uncertainty about how to gain access to the committee. If your committee has a low organizational profile, and there is no convenient way to contact a committee representative and receive a timely response, it is understandable why few requests for assistance are received.
- Inadequate committee representation. The size, diversity (including cultural and religious), and number of disciplines represented on your committee will certainly be related to your organization's size and mission, but the group should not be composed only of physicians and nurses. Restricting the membership in this way can bias perceptions of the committee's insight, credibility, and objectivity.

- Ineffectual leadership. As is true of any committee, the effectiveness of your ethics committee will often be directly related to the ability of its chairperson. Obviously, if this individual is disorganized, autocratic, or ingenuous, there will be fewer requests for consultation and other assistance.
- Insufficient organizational support. Although major funding is not required to facilitate a committee's activities, there must be a reasonable budget to cover the cost of publications and similar resources to support the continuing education of both committee members and stakeholders.
- Lack of initiative. A failure to develop and implement a creative strategic plan could be the most prevalent reason an ethics committee is underused and, as a result, marginally effective. Too many committees are simply passive and reactive, instead of pursuing a formal set of goals and objectives to maximize their value to the organizations they serve.

PRACTICAL STRATEGIES

To address your concern, you should first ask the committee to complete a comprehensive assessment of its performance. Such an audit should review the committee's purpose, composition, and activities. Begin by asking committee members to provide their assessment of the committee's:

1. Vision, values, and scope of services
2. Structure, authority, and relationship with other organizational entities
3. Frequency, convenience, and length of meetings; adequacy of agenda; and educational material
4. Process for evaluating its accomplishments, strengths, and weaknesses; communications within and outside the

organization; effectiveness of its policies and guidelines; and customer feedback

5. Success in defining and addressing its educational needs and those of the hospital community
6. Development, revision, and impact of ethical policies and guidelines
7. Resource support requirements
8. Case consultation process

After this self-assessment survey is completed and tabulated, you should share and discuss the results at the committee's annual retreat. It is likely that the group's annual goals and objectives will include preparing an action plan to address issues highlighted in the responses. Organizationwide surveys of past and potential committee users can also prove effective.

As mentioned, some committees have been asked to examine organizational ethics, and your committee could easily review the growing literature on this topic and initiate appropriate proposals or programs. Such an initiative might involve changing the scope of committee activities, its composition, and other aspects of its operation. Even if the number and magnitude of changes are relatively small, the organization, its staff, and patients will be the ultimate beneficiaries of a revitalized committee.

The practical strategies for the committee self-assessment come from Rebecca Dobbs' doctoral dissertation, which was recently submitted to Walden University in Minneapolis, MN.

Appendix A:
ACHE Code of Ethics*¹

Preface

The *Code of Ethics* is administered by the Ethics Committee, which is appointed by the Board of Governors upon nomination by the Chairman. It is composed of at least nine Diplomates or Fellows of the College, each of whom serves a three-year term on a staggered basis, with three members retiring each year.

The Ethics Committee shall:

- Review and evaluate annually the *Code of Ethics,* and make any necessary recommendations for updating the Code.
- Review and recommend action to the Board of Governors on allegations brought forth regarding breaches of the *Code of Ethics.*

---

*As amended by the Council of Regents at its annual meeting on March 25, 2000.
¹Appendices I and II, entitled "American College of Healthcare Executives Grievance Procedure" and "Ethics Committee Action," respectively, are a material part of this Code of Ethics and are incorporated herein by reference.

- Develop ethical policy statements to serve as guidelines of ethical conduct for healthcare executives and their professional relationships.
- Prepare an annual report of observations, accomplishments, and recommendations to the Board of Governors, and such other periodic reports as required.

The Ethics Committee invokes the *Code of Ethics* under authority of the ACHE *Bylaws*, Article II, Membership, Section 6, Resignation and Termination of Membership; Transfer to Inactive Status, subsection (b), as follows:

Membership may be terminated or rendered inactive by action of the Board of Governors as a result of violation of the *Code of Ethics;* nonconformity with the *Bylaws* or *Regulations Governing Admission, Advancement, Recertification, and Reappointment;* conviction of a felony; or conviction of a crime of moral turpitude or a crime relating to the healthcare management profession. No such termination of membership or imposition of inactive status shall be effected without affording a reasonable opportunity for the member to consider the charges and to appear in his or her own defense before the Board of Governors or its designated hearing committee, as outlined in the "Grievance Procedure," Appendix I of the College's *Code of Ethics.*

Preamble
The purpose of the *Code of Ethics* of the American College of Healthcare Executives is to serve as a guide to conduct for members. It contains standards of ethical behavior for healthcare executives in their professional relationships. These relationships include members of the healthcare executive's organization and other organizations.

Also included are patients or others served, colleagues, the community, and society as a whole. The *Code of Ethics* also incorporates standards of ethical behavior governing personal behavior, particularly when that conduct directly relates to the role and identity of the healthcare executive.

The fundamental objectives of the healthcare management profession are to enhance overall quality of life, dignity, and well-being of every individual needing healthcare services; and to create a more equitable, accessible, effective, and efficient healthcare system.

Healthcare executives have an obligation to act in ways that will merit the trust, confidence, and respect of healthcare professionals and the general public. Therefore, healthcare executives should lead lives that embody an exemplary system of values and ethics.

In fulfilling their commitments and obligations to patients or others served, healthcare executives function as moral advocates. Since every management decision affects the health and well-being of both individuals and communities, healthcare executives must carefully evaluate the possible outcomes of their decisions. In organizations that deliver healthcare services, they must work to safeguard and foster the rights, interests, and prerogatives of patients or others served. The role of moral advocate requires that healthcare executives speak out and take actions necessary to promote such rights, interests, and prerogatives if they are threatened.

I. **The healthcare executive's responsibilities to the profession of healthcare management**
    The healthcare executive shall:
    A. Uphold the values, ethics and mission of the healthcare management profession;
    B. Conduct all personal and professional activities with honesty, integrity, respect, fairness, and good faith in a manner that will reflect well upon the profession;

C. Comply with all laws pertaining to healthcare management in the jurisdictions in which the healthcare executive is located, or conducts professional activities;

D. Maintain competence and proficiency in healthcare management by implementing a personal program of assessment and continuing professional education;

E. Avoid the exploitation of professional relationships for personal gain;

F. Use this *Code* to further the interests of the profession and not for selfish reasons;

G. Respect professional confidences;

H. Enhance the dignity and image of the healthcare management profession through positive public information programs; and

I. Refrain from participating in any activity that demeans the credibility and dignity of the healthcare management profession.

II. **The healthcare executive's responsibilities to patients or others served, to the organization and employees**

A. *Responsibilities to Patients or Others Served*
The healthcare executive shall, within the scope of his or her authority:

1. Work to ensure the existence of a process to evaluate the quality of care or service rendered;

2. Avoid practicing or facilitating discrimination and institute safeguards to prevent discriminatory organizational practices;

3. Work to ensure the existence of a process that will advise patients or others served of the rights, opportunities, responsibilities, and risks regarding available healthcare services;

4. Work to provide a process that ensures the autonomy and self-determination of patients or others served; and

5. Work to ensure the existence of procedures that will safe-guard the confidentiality and privacy of patients or others served.

B. *Responsibilities to the Organization*
The healthcare executive shall, within the scope of his or her authority:

1. Provide healthcare services consistent with available resources and work to ensure the existence of a resource allocation process that considers ethical ramifications;

2. Conduct both competitive and cooperative activities in ways that improve community healthcare services;

3. Lead the organization in the use and improvement of standards of management and sound business practices;

4. Respect the customs and practices of patients or others served, consistent with the organization's philosophy; and

5. Be truthful in all forms of professional and organizational communication, and avoid disseminating information that is false, misleading, or deceptive.

C. *Responsibilities to Employees*
Healthcare executives have an ethical and professional obligation to employees of the organizations they manage that encompass but are not limited to:

1. Working to create a working environment conducive for underscoring employee ethical conduct and behavior;

2. Working to ensure that individuals may freely express ethical concerns and providing mechanisms for discussing and addressing such concerns;

3. Working to ensure a working environment that is free from harassment, sexual and other; coercion of any

kind, especially to perform illegal or unethical acts; and discrimination on the basis of race, creed, color, sex, ethnic origin, age or disability;

4. Working to ensure a working environment that is conducive to proper utilization of employees' skills and abilities;

5. Paying particular attention to the employee's work environment and job safety; and

6. Working to establish appropriate grievance and appeals mechanisms.

III. Conflicts of Interest

A conflict of interest may be only a matter of degree, but exists when the healthcare executive:

A. Acts to benefit directly or indirectly by using authority or inside information, or allows a friend, relative or associate to benefit from such authority or information.

B. Uses authority or information to make a decision to intentionally affect the organization in an adverse manner.

The healthcare executive shall:

A. Conduct all personal and professional relationships in such a way that all those affected are assured that management decisions are made in the best interests of the organization and the individuals served by it;

B. Disclose to the appropriate authority any direct or indirect financial or personal interests that pose potential or actual conflicts of interest;

C. Accept no gifts or benefits offered with the express or implied expectation of influencing a management decision; and

D. Inform the appropriate authority and other involved parties of potential or actual conflicts of interest related to appointments or elections to boards or committees inside or outside the healthcare executive's organization.

IV. **The healthcare executive's responsibilities to community and society**
The healthcare executive shall:
A. Work to identify and meet the healthcare needs of the community;
B. Work to ensure that all people have reasonable access to healthcare services;
C. Participate in public dialogue on healthcare policy issues and advocate solutions that will improve health status and promote quality healthcare;
D. Consider the short-term and long-term impact of management decisions on both the community and on society; and
E. Provide prospective consumers with adequate and accurate information, enabling them to make enlightened judgments and decisions regarding services.

V. **The healthcare executive's responsibility to report violations of the *Code***
A member of the College who has reasonable grounds to believe that another member has violated this *Code* has a duty to communicate such facts to the Ethics Committee.

Appendix I: American College of Healthcare Executives Grievance Procedure

1. In order to be processed by the College, a complaint must be filed in writing to the Ethics Committee of the College within

three years of the date of discovery of the alleged violation, and the Committee has the responsibility to look into incidents brought to its attention regardless of the informality of the information, provided the information can be documented or supported or may be a matter of public record. The three-year period within which a complaint must be filed shall temporarily cease to run during intervals when the accused member is in inactive status, or when the accused member resigns from the College.

2. The Committee chairman initially will determine whether the complaint falls within the purview of the Ethics Committee and whether immediate investigation is necessary. However, all letters of complaint that are filed with the Ethics Committee will appear on the agenda of the next committee meeting. The Ethics Committee shall have the final discretion to determine whether a complaint falls within the purview of the Ethics Committee.

3. If a grievance proceeding is initiated by the Ethics Committee:

   a. Specifics of the complaint will be sent to the respondent by certified mail. In such mailing, committee staff will inform the respondent that the grievance proceeding has been initiated, and that the respondent may respond directly to the Ethics Committee; the respondent also will be asked to cooperate with the Regent investigating the complaint.

   b. The Ethics Committee shall refer the matter to the appropriate Regent who is deemed best able to investigate the alleged infraction. The Regent shall make inquiry into the matter, and in the process the respondent shall be given an opportunity to be heard.

   c. Upon completion of the inquiry, the Regent shall present a complete report and recommended disposition of the matter in writing to the Ethics Committee. Absent unusual circumstances, the Regent is expected to complete his or her report and recommended disposition, and provide them to the Committee, within 60 days.

4. Upon the Committee's receipt of the Regent's report and recommended disposition, the Committee shall review them and make its written recommendation to the Board of Governors as to what action shall be taken and the reason or reasons therefor. A copy of the Committee's recommended decision along with the Regent's report and recommended disposition to the Board will be mailed to the respondent by certified mail. In such mailing, the respondent will be notified that within 30 days after his or her receipt of the Ethics Committee's recommended decision, the respondent may file a written appeal of the recommended decision with the Board of Governors.

5. Any written appeal submitted by the respondent must be received by the Board of Governors within 30 days after the recommended decision of the Ethics Committee is received by the respondent. The Board of Governors shall not take action on the Ethics Committee's recommended decision until the 30-day appeal period has elapsed. If no appeal to the Board of Governors is filed in a timely fashion, the Board shall review the recommended decision and determine action to be taken.

6. If an appeal to the Board of Governors is timely filed, the College Chairman shall appoint an ad hoc committee consisting of three Fellows to hear the matter. At least 30 days' notice of the formation of this committee, and of the hearing date, time and place, with an opportunity for representation, shall be mailed to the respondent. Reasonable requests for postponement shall be given consideration.

7. This ad hoc committee shall give the respondent adequate opportunity to present his or her case at the hearing, including the opportunity to submit a written statement and other documents deemed relevant by the respondent, and to be represented if so desired. Within a reasonable period of time

following the hearing, the ad hoc committee shall write a detailed report with recommendations to the Board of Governors.

8. The Board of Governors shall decide what action to take after reviewing the report of the ad hoc committee. The Board shall provide the respondent with a copy of its decision. The decision of the Board of Governors shall be final. The Board of Governors shall have the authority to accept or reject any of the findings or recommended decisions of the Regent, the Ethics Committee, or the ad hoc committee, and to order whatever level of discipline it feels is justified.

9. At each level of the grievance proceeding, the Board of Governors shall have the sole discretion to notify or contact the complainant relating to the grievance proceeding; provided, however, that the complainant shall be notified as to whether the complaint was reviewed by the Ethics Committee and whether the Ethics Committee or the Board of Governors has taken final action with respect to the complaint.

10. No individual shall serve on the ad hoc committee described above, or otherwise participate in these grievance proceedings on behalf of the College, if he or she is in direct economic competition with the respondent or otherwise has a financial conflict of interest in the matter, unless such conflict is disclosed to and waived in writing by the respondent.

11. All information obtained, reviewed, discussed, and otherwise used or developed in a grievance proceeding that is not otherwise publicly known, publicly available, or part of the public domain is considered to be privileged and strictly confidential information of the College, and is not to be disclosed to anyone outside of the grievance proceeding except as determined by the Board of Governors or as required by law; provided, however, that an individual's membership status is

not confidential and may be made available to the public upon request.

Appendix II: Ethics Committee Action

Once the grievance proceeding has been initiated, the Ethics Committee may take any of the following actions based upon its findings:

1. Determine the grievance complaint to be invalid.
2. Dismiss the grievance complaint.
3. Recommend censure.
4. Recommend transfer to inactive status for a specified minimum period of time.
5. Recommend expulsion.

Appendix B1: ACHE Ethical Policy Statement—Health Information Confidentiality

February 1994
November 1997 (revised)

Statement of the Issue

Healthcare is among the most personal services rendered in our society; yet to deliver this care, scores of personnel must have access to intimate patient information. In order to receive appropriate care, patients must feel free to reveal personal information. In return, the healthcare provider must offer patients confidentiality.

However, maintaining confidentiality is becoming more difficult. Information systems technology allows instant retrieval of medical information, widening access to a greater number of people. Within healthcare organizations, personal information contained in medical records is reviewed not only by physicians and nurses, but also by professionals in many clinical and administrative support areas.

Healthcare executives must follow the laws governing release of information. Releases cannot be made without proper authorization. Healthcare executives must determine that patients or their legal representatives consented to the release of information.

Some exceptions to patient confidentiality are necessary to promote public health, to protect children and spouses from abuse, and to comply with certain laws. Media representatives also seek access to health information, particularly when a patient is a public figure or when treatment involves legal or public health issues. Nevertheless, the rights of individual patients must be protected. Society's need for information rarely outweighs the right of patients to confidentiality.

Policy Position
The American College of Healthcare Executives believes that all healthcare executives have a moral and professional obligation to protect the confidentiality of patients' medical records. As patient advocates, executives must obtain proper patient authorization to release information or follow carefully defined policies on the release of information without consent.

While the healthcare organization owns the health record, the information in that record remains the patient's personal property. Organizations must determine the appropriateness of all requests for patient information and act accordingly.

In fulfilling their responsibilities, healthcare executives should seek to:

- Limit access to patient information to authorized individuals only.
- Ensure that institutional policies on confidentiality and release of information are consistent with regulations and laws.
- Educate healthcare personnel on confidentiality issues and take steps to ensure all healthcare personnel are aware of and understand their responsibilities to keep patient information confidential.
- Safeguard medical record files and computerized data with security and storage systems that protect against unauthorized access.

- Establish guidelines for masking patient identity in committee minutes and other working documents where the identity is not necessary.
- Ensure that policies concerning the right of patients to have access to their own medical records are clearly established and understood by appropriate staff.
- Create guidelines for securing necessary permissions for the release of medical information for research, education, utilization review, and other purposes.
- Adopt a specialized process to protect sensitive information such as psychiatric, HIV status, or substance abuse treatment records.
- Identify special situations that require consultation with senior management prior to release of information.
- When appropriate, seek written agreements that detail the obligations of confidentiality for individuals and agencies who receive medical records information.
- Collaborate with media representatives to develop procedures for the request of and release of medical information about patients in the public domain.
- Educate patients about organizational policies on confidentiality.
- Participate in the public dialogue on confidentiality issues such as employer use of healthcare information and public health reporting.

The American College of Healthcare Executives urges all healthcare executives to maintain an appropriate balance between the patient's right to confidentiality and the need to release information in the public's interest.

Approved by the Board of Governors on November 2, 1997.

Appendix B2: ACHE Ethical Policy Statement—Ethical Decision Making for Healthcare Executives

August 1993
February 1997 (revised)

Statement of the Issue

Many factors have contributed to the growing concern in healthcare organizations with ethical issues, includingpressure to reduce costs, mergers and acquisitions, financialand other resource constraints, and advances in medicaltechnology that complicate decision-making near the end of life. Healthcare executives have a responsibility to address the growing number of complex ethical dilemmas they are facing, but they cannot and should not make such decisions alone or without a sound decision-making framework. Healthcare organizations should have vehicles, such as ethics committees, conflict-of-interest statements, written policies and procedures, and/or a staff ethicist, to assist healthcare executives with the decision-making process. With these and other appropriate organizational mechanisms, the sometimes conflicting interests of patients, families, physicians and other caregivers, payors, the organization, and the community can be appropriately weighed and balanced.

Policy Position

The American College of Healthcare Executives believes educational training in ethics is an important step in a healthcare executive's lifelong commitment to high ethical conduct, both personally and professionally. Further, the College supports the development of organizational mechanisms that enable healthcare executives to appropriately and expeditiously address ethical dilemmas. The College encourages its members as leaders in their organizations and the communities their organizations serve, to take an active role in the development and ongoing use of these organizational mechanisms. Further, it is incumbent upon healthcare executives to lead in a manner that sets an ethical tone for their organizations. To this end, healthcare executives should:

- Communicate the organization's commitment to ethical decision making through its mission and value statements and/or organizational code of ethics.
- Develop organizational mechanisms that are flexible enough to deal with the spectrum of ethical concerns—medical, social, financial—and address them within the context of their organizations' mission and values. Whereas physicians, nurses, and other caregivers may primarily address ethical issues on a case-by-case basis, healthcare executives have a responsibility to also address those issues with broader community and societal implications.
- Organizational mechanisms, therefore, must facilitate ethical decision making as it relates to the spectrum of issues ranging from the allocation of scarce resources to patient-specific ethical issues.
- Promote organizational mechanisms that allow for diverse input. An organization's ethics committee, for example, might include physicians, nurses, managers, board members, social workers, attorneys, patient and/or community representatives,

and the clergy. All of these groups are likely to bring unique and valuable perspectives to bear on discussions of ethical issues.

- Evaluate and continually refine organizational processes for addressing ethical issues. Beyond the creation of an ethics committee, healthcare executives should consider developing ethical standards of conduct and offering educational programming to boards, staff, physicians, and others on these standards and on the more global issues of ethical decision making in today's healthcare environment. Further, healthcare executives should promote learning opportunities, such as those provided through professional society involvement or undergraduate and graduate health administration programs, that will facilitate open discussion of ethical issues.

- Promote decision making that results in the appropriate use of power, protection of human rights, and consideration of organizational and societal issues. To this end, healthcare executives must take the lead in raising difficult issues; educating; presenting options; demonstrating personal, professional, and organizational integrity; and encouraging societal solutions to ethical dilemmas.

No one organizational mechanism or policy will be universally effective. Each organization, under the leadership of its executives, must develop its own processes and procedures for discussing and resolving such sensitive issues.

Approved by the Board of Governors of the American College of Healthcare Executives on February 28, 1997.

Appendix B3: ACHE Ethical Policy Statement—Creating an Ethical Environment for Employees

March 1992
August 1995 (revised)
November 2000 (revised)

Statement of the Issue

The number and magnitude of challenges facing healthcare organizations are unprecedented. Growing financial pressures, rising public and payor expectations, and the increasing number of consolidations have placed hospitals, health networks, managed care plans, and other healthcare organizations under greater stress-thus potentially intensifying ethical dilemmas.

Now, more than ever, the healthcare organization must be managed with consistently high professional and ethical standards. This means that the executive, acting with other responsible parties, must support an environment conducive not only to providing high quality, cost-effective healthcare, but which also encourages individual ethical development. The executive must also support and implement a systematic approach to training related to corporate compliance for all staff.

The ability of an organization to achieve its full potential will remain dependent upon the motivation and skills of its staff. Thus, the executive has an obligation to accomplish the organization's mission in a manner that respects the values of individuals and maximizes their contributions.

Policy Position
The American College of Healthcare Executives believes that all healthcare executives have an ethical and professional obligation to employees of the organizations they manage to create a working environment that supports, but is not limited to:

- Responsible employee ethical conduct and behavior;
- Free expression of ethical concerns and mechanisms for discussing and addressing such concerns without retribution;
- Use of a hotline or other approach that safeguards employees who wish to raise ethical concerns;
- Freedom from all harassment, coercion, and discrimination;
- Appropriate utilization of an employee's skills and abilities;
- A safe work environment.

These responsibilities can best be implemented in an environment where all employees are encouraged to develop the highest standards of ethics. This should be done with attention to other features of the Code of Ethics, particularly those that stress the moral character of the executive and the organization itself.

Approved by the Board of Governors of the American College of Healthcare Executives on November 13, 2000.

Appendix B4: ACHE Ethical Policy Statement—Impaired Healthcare Executives

February 1991
March 1995 (revised)
November 2000 (revised)

Statement of the Issue

The American College of Healthcare Executives recognizes that impairment in the form of alcoholism, substance abuse, chemical dependency, mental/emotional instability, or senility is a problem the affects all of society. Substance abuse is a pervasive problem in today's society, affecting individuals of all ages and in all walks of life. Mental/emotional instability and senility are also problems that cross all boundaries in society.

Impaired healthcare executives affect not only themselves and their families, but they also have a significant impact on their profession; their professional society; their organizations, colleagues, patients, clients, and others served; their communities; and society as a whole. Impairment typically leads to misconduct in the form of incompetence and unsafe or unprofessional behavior, which can also lead to substantial costs associated with loss of productivity and errors in judgment.

The impaired healthcare executive can damage the public image of his or her organization of employment. Public confidence in the organization diminishes if it appears that the organization is not being managed with consistently high standards of professional and ethical practice. This lack of public confidence may cause the community to deem the organization unworthy of its support.

Society expects healthcare executives to practice the standards of good health that they advocate for the public. Impaired healthcare executives diminish the credibility of the profession and its ability to manage society's healthcare when they are not appropriately managing their own personal health.

Policy Position

The preamble of the American College of Healthcare Executives Code of Ethics states that "healthcare executives have an obligation to act in ways that will merit the trust, confidence, and respect of healthcare professionals and the general public. To do this, healthcare executives must lead lives that embody an exemplary system of values and ethics."

The American College of Healthcare Executives believes that all healthcare executives have an ethical and a professional obligation to:

- Maintain a personal health status that is free from impairment.
- Refrain from all professional activities if impaired.
- Expeditiously seek treatment if impairment occurs.
- Urge impaired colleagues to expeditiously seek treatment and to refrain from all professional activities while impaired.
- Report the impairment to the appropriate person or persons, should the colleague refuse to seek professional assistance and should the state of impairment persist.
- Recommend or provide, within one's employing organization, avenues for reporting impairment and either access or referral to treatment or assistance programs.

- Urge the community to provide information and resources for assistance and treatment of alcoholism, substance abuse, mental/emotional instability, and senility as needed and appropriate.

Approved by the Board of Governors of the American College of Healthcare Executives on November 13, 2000.

Appendix B5: ACHE Ethical Policy Statement—Decisions Near the End of Life

August 1994
November 1999 (revised)

Statement of the Issue

Medical technology has shaped the circumstances of death, giving us options about when, where, and how we die. Intervening at the moment of death, technology can now sustain lives, but often there is little or no hope for recovery or for a meaningful existence.

Fearful of economic dependency and loss of self, patients and/or proxies are exercising more influence over decisions near the end of life. The traditional value to preserve life by all possible means is now being weighed against quality-of-life considerations.

Policy Position

The American College of Healthcare Executives urges healthcare executives to address the ethical dilemmas and problems surrounding death and promote public dialog that will lead to awareness and resolution of death with dignity concerns.

ACHE encourages all healthcare executives to play a significant role in addressing this issue:

- Healthcare executives should advocate the completion of advance directives, including living wills and durable powers of attorney for healthcare. Ideally, such documents should be prepared prior to hospitalization or a medical crisis.
- These and similar legal mechanisms encourage people to consider under what circumstances they would not want certain life-prolonging treatments. Use of a power of attorney or laws that permit the appointment of a proxy have the added advantage of allowing individuals to designate a specific person who would make treatment choices for them at any time they lack decision-making capacity. The ultimate objective of advance directives is to protect the rights of patients to influence clinical decisions affecting their care.
- Healthcare executives have a responsibility to ensure their organizations provide support for patients and their families as treatment decisions are reached. Patient autonomy (the right of an individual to influence decision affecting his or her treatment) should remain at the core of this process.
- When there is disagreement on treatment for incompetent patients (even those patients who have valid advance directives or a durable power of attorney), the guidance of an ethics committee or similar resource may aid in resolution. Healthcare executives should develop clear guidelines to handle disputes and provide support to physicians and families responsible for making treatment choices.
- When developing and implementing guidelines, healthcare executives must encourage cooperation and understanding of ethical decision making among members of the governing body, executive management, physicians, and other members of the healthcare team. Executives should work to develop methods of raising awareness and providing education regarding sensitivity to ethical dilemmas.

- Executives should heighten awareness of ethical issues surrounding the right to choose treatment through information forums that promote open discussion among patients and their families, attorneys, clergy, journalists, physicians, and other healthcare professionals. By raising moral and ethical questions, healthcare executives will aid the public in understanding the growing impact of technology on death and dying.

Healthcare executives must foster reasoned, compassionate decision making that considers the rights and values of patients and staff. While interpretation of these principles will vary by local custom and law, healthcare executives have a responsibility to ensure that their organizations operate with respond for the inherent worth and human dignity of every individual.

Approved by the Board of Governors of the American College of Healthcare Executives on November 15, 1999.

Appendix B6: ACHE Ethical Policy Statement—Ethical Issues Related to a Reduction in Force

August 1995
November 2000 (revised)

Statement of the Issue

As the result of managed care, declining admissions, shorter lengths of stay, higher productivity, new technology, and other factors, the capacity of many healthcare organizations exceeds demand. Consequently, a large number of organizations will reduce their work forces. Additionally, mergers and consolidations will result in further reductions and reassignments of staff. Financial pressures will continue to fuel this trend. However, patient care needs should not be compromised when determining staffing requirements.

The hardship and stress of a reduction in force can be lessened by careful planning, cost management, resource management, growth focus, and proactive management of human resources. Formal policies and procedures should be developed well in advance of the need to implement them.

The decision to reduce staff necessitates consideration of the short-term and long-term impact on all employees—those leaving and those remaining. Decision makers should consider the potential ethical conflict between formally stated organizational values and their reduction actions.

Policy Position
The American College of Healthcare Executives recommends that specific steps be considered by healthcare executives when initiating a reduction in force process to support consistency between stated organizational values and those demonstrated during and after the process. Among these steps are the following:

- Provide timely, accurate, clear, and consistent information to the stakeholders when staff reductions become necessary;
- Review values expressed in mission and value statements, personnel policies, annual reports, employee orientation material, and other documents to test congruence and conformance with reduction in force actions;
- Support, through retraining and redeployment, if possible, employees whose positions have been eliminated. Also, consider outplacement assistance and appropriate severance policies, if possible; and
- Address the needs of remaining staff by demonstrating sensitivity to their potential feelings of loss, anger, and survivor guilt. Also address their anxiety about the possibility of further reductions, uncertainty regarding changes in work load and work redesign, and other similar concerns.

Healthcare organizations encounter the same set of challenging issues associated with reductions in force as do other employers. Reduction in force decisions should reflect ethical values.

Approved by the Board of Governors of the American College of Healthcare Executives on November 13, 2000.

Appendix C: ACHE Ethics Self-Assessment Instrument

How to Use this Self-Assessment

All affiliates of the American College of Healthcare Executives agree, as a condition of membership, to abide by ACHE's *Code of Ethics*. But in a rapidly changing marketplace characterized by mounting challenges, new relationships, and rapid technological change, even the best-intentioned healthcare executive is likely to struggle with certain ethical dilemmas.

This self-assessment is designed to help you identify those areas where you are on strong ethical ground; areas where you may wish to examine the basis for your responses; and opportunities for further reflection. *This tool is intended for personal use and should not be returned to ACHE.* In addition, it should not be considered a tool for evaluating others' ethical behavior.

We hope that you find this self-assessment thought-provoking and useful. You are to be commended for taking time out of your hectic schedule to complete it.

After You've Completed the Self-Assessment

Once you have finished the self-assessment, it is suggested that you review your responses, noting which questions you answered "usually," "occasionally," and "almost never." You may find that in some cases, an answer of "usually" is satisfactory, but in other cases, such as when answering a question about protecting staff's well-being, an answer of "usually" may raise an "ethical red flag." You will note that the instrument does not have a scoring mechanism; this is intentional. We do not believe that ethical behavior can or should be quantified.

We are confident that you will uncover few red flags and that if you do, you will willingly and appropriately address them. We also want you to consider your professional society as an additional resource when you and your management team are confronted with difficult ethical dilemmas. For example, you can refer to our regular "Healthcare Management Ethics" column in *Healthcare Executive* magazine as well as ACHE's *Ethical Policy Statements.*

Please circle one answer for each of the following questions.

Almost Never: AN   Occassionally: O   Usually: U
Always: A   Not Applicable: NA

I. LEADERSHIP

I take courageous, consistent, and appropriate management actions to overcome barriers to achieving my organization's mission.	AN O U A NA
I place community/patient benefit over my personal gain.	AN O U A NA
I work to ensure that decisions about access to care are based primarily on medical necessity, not only on the ability to pay.	AN O U A NA
My statements and actions are consistent with a professional standard of propriety.	AN O U A NA
My statements and actions are honest even when circumstances would allow me to confuse the issues.	AN O U A NA
I advocate ethical decision making by the board, management team, and medical staff.	AN O U A NA

I encourage innovative actions as appropriate,   AN   O   U   A   NA
even when maintaining the status quo would be
an easier choice.

I use an ethically sensitive approach to conflict   AN   O   U   A   NA
resolution.

I initiate and encourage discussion of the ethical   AN   O   U   A   NA
aspects of management/financial issues.

I initiate and promote discussion of controversial   AN   O   U   A   NA
issues affecting community/patient health, e.g.,
domestic and community violence and decisions
near the end of life.

I promptly and candidly explain to internal and   AN   O   U   A   NA
external stakeholders negative economic trends
and encourage appropriate action.

I use my authority solely to fulfill my responsi-   AN   O   U   A   NA
bilities and not for self-interest or to further the
interests of family, friends, or associates.

When an ethical dilemma confronts my organiza-   AN   O   U   A   NA
tion or me, I am successful in finding an effective
resolution process and ensuring it is followed.

I demonstrate respect for my colleagues, superiors,   AN   O   U   A   NA
and staff.

I demonstrate that my organization's vision,   AN   O   U   A   NA
mission, and value statements are living
documents.

I make timely decisions rather than delaying them   AN   O   U   A   NA
to avoid difficult or politically risky choices.

My personal expense reports are accurate and are   AN   O   U   A   NA
only billed to a single organization.

Community

I promote community health status improvement   AN   O   U   A   NA
as a guiding goal of my organization and as a
cornerstone of my efforts on behalf of my
organization.

I personally devote time to developing solutions   AN   O   U   A   NA
to community health problems.

I encourage my management team to devote   AN   O   U   A   NA
personal time to community service.

Patients and Their Families

I am a patient advocate on both clinical and   AN   O   U   A   NA
financial matters.

I ensure equitable treatment of patients regardless   AN   O   U   A   NA
of socioeconomic group or payor category.

I demonstrate through organizational policies   AN   O   U   A   NA
and personal actions that overtreatment and
undertreatment of patients are unacceptable.

I protect patients' rights to autonomy, clinical   AN   O   U   A   NA
efficacy, and full information about their illnesses,
treatment options, and related costs.

I promote medical record confidentiality and do   AN   O   U   A   NA
not tolerate breaches of this confidentiality.

Board

I have a system in place for board members to   AN   O   U   A   NA
make full disclosure and reveal potential conflicts
of interest.

I ensure that reports to the board, my own or   AN O U A NA
others', appropriately convey risks of decisions
or proposed projects.

I work to keep the board focused on ethical issues   AN O U A NA
of importance to the community and other
stakeholders.

I promote board discussion of resource allocation   AN O U A NA
issues, particularly those where organizational
and community interests may appear to be
incompatible.

I keep the board appropriately informed about   AN O U A NA
issues of alleged financial malfeasance, clinical
malpractice, and potential litigious situations
involving employees.

Colleagues and Staff

I maintain confidences entrusted to me.   AN O U A NA

I demonstrate through personal actions and   AN O U A NA
organizational policies zero tolerance for any
form of staff harassment.

I fulfill the promises I make.   AN O U A NA

I am respectful of views different from mine.   AN O U A NA

I am respectful of individuals who differ from me   AN O U A NA
in ethnicity, gender, education, or job position.

I convey negative news promptly and openly, not   AN O U A NA
allowing employees or others to be misled.

I promote professional development for staff, for   AN O U A NA
their benefit and the benefit of the organization.

I demonstrate that incompetent supervision is not tolerated and make timely decisions regarding marginally performing managers.

AN O U A NA

My staffing plan minimizes the need for sudden layoffs or other crisis-driven responses to external financial pressures.

AN O U A NA

I ensure adherence to policies affecting staff.

AN O U A NA

I am sensitive to employees who have ethical concerns and facilitate resolution of these concerns.

AN O U A NA

I act quickly and decisively when employees are not treated fairly in their relationships with other employees.

AN O U A NA

I assign staff only to official duties and do not ask them to assist me with work on behalf of my family, friends, or associates.

AN O U A NA

I hold all staff and clinical/business partners accountable for compliance with professional standards, including ethical behavior.

AN O U A NA

Clinicians

When problems arise with clinical care, I ensure that the problems receive prompt attention and resolution by the responsible parties.

AN O U A NA

I insist that my organization's clinical practice guidelines are consistent with our vision, mission, and value statements.

AN O U A NA

When variations in care suggest quality of care is at stake, I encourage timely actions that serve patients' interests.

AN O U A NA

I insist that participating clinicians and staff live   AN   O   U   A   NA
up to the terms of managed care contracts.

I encourage resource allocation that is equitable, is   AN   O   U   A   NA
based on clinical needs, and appropriately balances
patient needs and organizational/clinical resources.

I expeditiously and forthrightly deal with impaired   AN   O   U   A   NA
clinicians and take necessary action when I believe
a clinician is not competent to perform his/her
clinical duties.

Buyers, Payors, and Vendors

I negotiate, and expect my management team to   AN   O   U   A   NA
negotiate, in good faith.

I personally disclose, and expect board members,   AN   O   U   A   NA
staff members, and clinicians to disclose, any
possible conflicts of interests before pursuing or
entering into relationships with potential business
partners.

I set an example for others in my organization by   AN   O   U   A   NA
not accepting personal gifts from vendors.

Appendix D: Ethics Resources

Journals

The American Journal of Bioethics (MIT Press)

Bioethics Forum (Princeton University)

Cambridge Quarterly of Healthcare Ethics (Cambridge University Press)

Hastings Center Report (The Hastings Center)

IRB: A Review of Human Subjects Research (The Hastings Center)

HEC (HealthCare Ethics Committee) Forum (Kluwer Online)

Journal of Business Ethics

Journal of Clinical Ethics (University Publishing Group)

Journal of Law, Medicine, and Ethics (American Society of Law, Medicine & Ethics)

Journal of Religious Ethics (Blackwell Publishers)

Kennedy Institute of Ethics (The Johns Hopkins University Press)

Philosophy and Public Affairs (The Johns Hopkins University Press)

Theoretical Medicine (Kluwer Academic Publishers)

Organizations
American Society for Bioethics and Humanities
4700 W. Lake Avenue
Glenview, IL 60025
(847) 375-4745

American Society of Law, Medicine & Ethics
765 Commonwealth Avenue, 16th floor
Boston, MA 02215
(617) 262-4990

Centers
Bioethics Forum (Princeton University)
Bioethics Institute (Johns Hopkins University)
Bioethics Institute (New York Medical College)
Bioethics Program (Iowa State University)
Center for Bioethics (University of Minnesota)
Center for Bioethics (University of Pennsylvania)
Center for Bioethics and Health Law (University of Pittsburgh)
Center for Biomedical Ethics (Case Western Reserve
  University)
Center for Biomedical Ethics (University of Virginia)
Center for Biomedical Ethics (Stanford University)
Center for Christian Bioethics (Loma Linda University)
Center for Clinical Ethics and Humanities in Health Care
  (University of Buffalo)
Center for Clinical and Research Ethics (Vanderbilt University)
Center for Ethics in Health Care (Oregon Health Sciences
  University)
Center for Ethics and Humanities in the Life Sciences
  (Michigan State University)
Center for Health Care Ethics (St. Louis University)
Center for Health Ethics and Law (West Virginia University)

Center for Health Ethics and Policy (University of Colorado, Denver)
Center for Medical Ethics and Health Policy (Baylor University)
Center for the Study of Bioethics (Medical College of Wisconsin)
Center for the Study of Medical Ethics Humanities (Duke University)
Center for the Study of Society and Medicine (Columbia University)
Consortium Ethics Program (University of Pittsburgh)
Division of Medical Ethics (University of Utah)
Department of Medical Humanities and Bioethics Center (East Carolina University)
Department of Bioethics (Cleveland Clinic Foundation)
Ethics in Medicine (University of Washington)
Forum for Bioethics and Philosophy (University of Miami)
The Hastings Center (Garrison, New York)
Institute for Business and Professional Ethics (DePaul University)
Institute for Jewish Medical Ethics (San Francisco)
Institute for Ethics (American Medical Association)
Institute for Medical Humanities (University of Texas Medical Branch)
Institute for the Study of Applied and Professional Ethics (Dartmouth College)
Kennedy Institute of Ethics (Georgetown University)
Maclean Center for Clinical Medical Ethics (University of Chicago)
Markkula Center for Applied Ethics (Santa Clara University)
Medical Humanities and Bioethics Department (East Carolina University)
Midwest Bioethics Center (Kansas City, Missouri)
National Bioethics Advisory Commission (Rockville, Maryland)

National Center for Ethics (Veterans Health Administration,
White River Junction, Vermont)
Neiswanger Institute of Bioethics and Health Policy (Loyola
University Medical Center)
Park Ridge Center (Chicago)
Program in Ethics and the Professions (Harvard University)
Program in Society and Medicine (University of Michigan
Medical Center)

Web Sites

http://www.ama-assn.org/sitemap.htm
America Medical Association Council on Medical and Judicial
Affairs

http://www.asbh.org
American Society for Bioethics and Humanities

http://www.aslme.org
American Society of Law, Medicine, & Ethics

http://www.bioethics.net
Center for Bioethics (University of Pennsylvania)

http://www.pitt.edu/~bioethic/
Center for Bioethics and Health Law (University of
Pittsburgh)

http://onlineethics.org/text/glossary.html
Center for Biomedical Ethics (Case Western Reserve
University)

http://www.stanford.edu/dept/scbe/
Center for Biomedical Ethics (Stanford University)

http://www.med.virginia.edu/bioethics
Center for Biomedical Ethics (University of Virginia)

http://www.mcw.edu/bioethics/
Center for the Study of Bioethics (Medical College of
  Wisconsin)

http://bioethics.georgetown.edu
Kennedy Institute of Ethics

http://www.bioethics.gov
National Bioethics Advisory Commission

http://www.va.gov/ethics
National Center for Ethics

http://www.epistemelinks.com
philosophical resources

Selected Bibliography

General References

American College of Physicians. 1998. "Ethics Manual, 4th ed." *Annals of Internal Medicine* 128 (7): 576–594.

American Hospital Association. 1994. *Values in Conflict: Ethical Issues in Health Care, 2nd ed.* Chicago: American Hospital Association.

Catholic Health Association. 1991. *Corporate Ethics in Healthcare.* St. Louis, MO: Catholic Health Association.

Darr, K. 1995. *Ethics in Health Services Management, 2nd ed.* Baltimore, MD: Health Professions Press.

deGeorge, R. 1995. *Business Ethics, 4th ed.* New York: Macmillan.

Devettere, R. 2000. *Practical Decision Making in Health Care Ethics: Cases and Concepts, 2nd ed.* Washington, DC: Georgetown University Press.

Frankena, W. 1973. *Ethics.* Englewood Cliffs, NJ: Prentice Hall.

Freeman, R. (editor). 1991. *Business Ethics: The State of the Art.* New York: Oxford University Press.

Friedman, E. (editor). 1992. *Choices and Conflict: Explorations in Health Care Ethics.* Chicago: American Hospital Association.

———. 1996. *The Right Thing: Ten Years of Ethics Columns from the Healthcare Forum Journal.* San Francisco: Jossey-Bass.

Garrett, T., H. Baillie, and R. Garrett. 1989. *Health Care Ethics: Principles and Problems.* Englewood Cliffs, NJ: Prentice Hall.

Grafius, L. 1995. *Ethics for Everyone: A Practical Guide to Interdisciplinary Biomedical Ethics Education.* Chicago: American Hospital Publishing Inc.

Griffith, J. 1993. *The Moral Challenges of Health Care Management.* Chicago: Health Administration Press.

Hiller, M. 1986. *Ethics and Health Administration: Ethical Decision Making in Health Management.* Arlington, TX: Association of University Programs in Health Administration.

Kuczewski, M., and R. Pinkus. 1999. *An Ethics Casebook for Hospitals: Practical Approaches to Everyday Cases.* Washington, DC: Georgetown University Press.

MacIntyre, A. 1984. *After Virtue.* Notre Dame, IN: Notre Dame University Press.

Macklin, R. 1987. *Mortal Choices: Ethical Dilemmas in Modern Medicine.* Boston: Howard Mifflin Company.

Rachels, J. 1982. "Can Ethics Provide Answers?" *Hastings Center Report* 12 (3): 32–40.

Reich W. 1995. *Encyclopedia of Bioethics (Revised Edition).* New York: MacMillan, Simon & Schuster.

Reiser, S. 1994. "The Ethical Life of Health Care Organizations." *Hastings Center Report* 24 (6): 28–35.

Spencer, E., A. Mills, M. Rorty, and P. Werhane. 2000. *Organization Ethics in Health Care.* New York: Oxford Press.

Stark, A. 1993. "What's the Matter with Business Ethics?" *Harvard Business Review* 71 (3): 38–48.

Tamborini-Martin, S., and K. Hanley. 1989. "The Importance of Being Ethical." *Health Progress* 70 (5): 24–27, 82.

Warnock, G. 1993. "The Object of Morality." *Cambridge Quarterly of Healthcare Ethics* 2 (3): 255–258.

Werhane, P. 1990. "The Ethics of Health Care as a Business." *Business & Professional Ethics Journal* 9 (3 & 4): 7–20.

Woodstock Theological Center. 1995. *Ethical Considerations in the Business Aspects of Health Care.* Washington: Georgetown University Press.

Worthley, J. A. 1997. *The Ethics of the Ordinary in Healthcare: Concepts and Cases*. Chicago: Health Administration Press.

Managed Care

Agich, G., and H. Foster. 2000. Conflicts of Interest and Management in Managed Care. *Cambridge Quarterly of Healthcare Ethics* 9 (2): 189–204.

Council on Ethical and Judicial Affairs. 1995. "Ethical Issues in Managed Care." *Journal of the American Medical Association* 273 (4): 330–335.

Emanuel, E. 2000. "Justice and Managed Care: Four Principles for the Just Allocation of Health Care Resources." *Hastings Center Report* 30 (3): 8–16.

Friedman, L., and G. Savage. 1998. "Can Ethical Management and Managed Care Coexist?" *Health Care Management Review* 23 (2): 56–62.

Greene, J. 1997. "Has Managed Care Lost Its Soul?" *Hospitals & Health Networks* 71 (10): 36–42.

Howe, E. 1995. "Managed Care: New Moves, Moral Uncertainty, and a Radical Attitude." *Journal of Clinical Ethics* 6 (4): 290–371.

Jacobson, P., and M. Cahill. 2000. "Applying Fiduciary Responsibilities in the Managed Care Context." *American Journal of Law, Medicine & Ethics* 26 (2 & 3): 155–173.

Khushf, G. 1999. "The Case for Managed Care." *Journal of Medicine and Philosophy* 24 (5): 415–550.

Morreim, E. 1995. *Balancing Act: The New Medical Ethics of Medicine's New Economics*. Washington, DC: Georgetown University Press.

———. 1999. "Assessing Quality of Care: New Twists from Managed Care." *Journal of Clinical Ethics* 10 (2): 88–99.

Paris, J., and S. Post. 2000. "Managed Care, Cost Control, and the Common Good." *Cambridge Quarterly of Healthcare Ethics* 9 (2): 182–188.

Perkel, R. 1996. "Ethics and Managed Care." *Medical Clinics of North America* 80 (2): 263–278.

Veatch, R. 1997. "Who Should Manage Care? The Care for Patients." *Kennedy Institute of Ethics Journal* 7 (4): 391–401.

Veatch, R., and C. Spicer. 1997. "Ethical Challenges in Managed Care." *Kennedy Institute of Ethics Journal* 7 (4).

Cost Containment and Resource Allocation

Asch, D., and P. Ubel. 1997. "Rationing by Any Other Name." *New England Journal of Medicine* 336 (23): 1668–1671.

Boyle, P., and E. Moskowitz. 1996. "Making Tough Resource Decisions." *Health Progress* 77 (6): 48–53.

Buchanan, A. 1998. "Managed Care: Rationing Without Justice, But Not Unjustly." *Journal of Health Politics, Policy, and Law* 23 (4): 617–634.

Callahan, D. 2000. "Rationing, Equity, and Affordable Care." *Health Progress* 81 (4): 38–41.

Cochran, C., J. Kupersmith, and T. McGovern. 2000. "Justice, Allocation, and Managed Care." *Health Progress* 81 (4): 34–37, 41.

Daniels, N. 1986. "Why Saying No to Patients in the United States Is so Hard: Cost Containment, Justice, and Provider Autonomy." *New England Journal of Medicine* 314 (21): 1380–1383.

Grumbach, K., and T. Bodenheimer. 1994. "Painful vs. Painless Cost Control." *Journal of the American Medical Association* 272 (18): 1458–1464.

Powers, M., and R. Faden. 2000. "Inequalities in Health. Inequalities in Healthcare: Four Generations of Discussion About Justice and Cost-Effectiveness Analysis." *Kennedy Institute of Ethics Journal* 10 (2): 109–127.

Ethics Committees and Consultation

American Society for Bioethics and Humanities. 1998. "Core Competencies for Healthcare Ethics Consultation." Glenview, IL: ASBH.

Aulisio, M., R. Arnold, and S. Youngner. 2000. "Health Care Ethics Consultation: Nature, Goals, and Competencies." *Annals of Internal Medicine* 133 (1): 59–69.

Harding, J. 1994. "The Role of Organizational Ethics Committees." *Physician Executive* 20 (2): 19–24.

Hirsch, N. 1999. "All in the Family—Siblings but not Twins: The Relationship of Clinical and Organizational Ethics Analysis." *Journal of Clinical Ethics* 10 (3): 187–193.

Lawry, T. 1999. "Ethicists Have Gone Digital." *Health Progress* 80 (5): 10–11.

McCullough, L. 1998. "Preventive Ethics, Managed Practice, and the Hospital Ethics Committee as a Resource for Physician Executives." *Healthcare Ethics Committee Forum* 10 (2): 136–151.

Myser, C., P. Donehower, and C. Frank. 1999. "Making the Most of Disequilibrium: Bridging the Gap Between Clinical and Organizational Ethics in a Newly Merged Healthcare Organization." *Journal of Clinical Ethics* 10 (3): 194–201.

Nelson W., and G. Wlody. 1999. "The Evolving Role of Ethics Advisory Committees in VHA." *Healthcare Ethics Committee Forum* 9 (2): 129–146.

Potter, R. 1996. "From Clinical Ethics to Organizational Ethics: The Second Stage of the Evolution of Bioethics." *Bioethics Forum* 12 (2): 3–12.

———. 1999. "On Our Way to Integrated Bioethics: Clinical/Organizational/Communal." *Journal of Clinical Ethics* 10 (2): 171–177.

Renz, D., and W. Eddy. 1996. "Organizations, Ethics, and Health Care: Building an Ethics Infrastructure for a New Era." *Bioethics Forum* 12 (2): 29–39.

Spencer, E. 1997. "A New Role for Institutional Ethics Committees: Organizational Ethics." *Journal of Clinical Ethics* 8 (4): 372–376.

Leadership

Badaracco, J., and R. Ellsworth. 1989. *Leadership and the Quest for Integrity.* Boston: Harvard Business School Press.

Fenner, K., and M. Basford. 1999. "How Can Leaders Ensure Organizational Integrity?" *Trustee* 52 (3): 26–27.

Lombardi, D. 1997. *Reorganization and Renewal: Strategies for Healthcare Leaders.* Chicago: Health Administration Press.

Clinical Care Issues

Berger, J., and F. Rosener. 1996. "The Ethics of Practice Guidelines." *Archives of Internal Medicine* 156 (18): 2051–2056.

Howe, E. 1999. "Organizational Ethics' Greatest Challenges: Factoring in Less-Reachable Patients." *Journal of Clinical Ethics* 10 (4): 263–270.

————. 2000. "Leaving Luputa: What Doctors Aren't Taught About Informed Consent." *Journal of Clinical Ethics* 11 (1): 3–13.

Levinsky, N. 1996. "Social, Institutional, and Economic Barriers to the Exercise of Patients' Rights." *New England Journal of Medicine* 334 (8): 532–534.

Mazur, D. 2001. *Shared Decision Making in the Patient-Physician Relationship: Challenges Facing Patients, Physicians, and Medical Institutions.* Tampa, FL: American College of Physician Executives.

O'Toole, B. 1998. "Four Ways People Approach Ethics." *Health Progress* 79 (6): 38–41, 43.

Pellegrino, E. 1997. "Managed Care at the Bedside: How Do We Look in the Moral Mirror?" *Kennedy Institute of Ethics Journal* 7 (4): 321–330.

Rhodes, R. "Futility and the Goals of Medicine." *Journal of Clinical Ethics* 9 (2): 194–205.

Smith, M., and H. Forster. 2000. "Morally Managing Medical Mistakes." *Cambridge Quarterly of Healthcare Ethics* 9 (1): 38–53.

Solovy, A. 1999. "The Price of Dignity." *Hospitals & Health Networks* 73 (3): 30.

Woolf, S. 1999. "The Need For Perspective in Evidence-Based Medicine." *Journal of the American Medical Association* 282 (24): 2358–2365.

Organizational and Management Issues

Blake, D. 1999. "Organizational Ethics: Creating Structural and Cultural Change in Healthcare Organizations." *The Journal of Clinical Ethics* 10 (3): 187–193.

Brett, A., J. Raymond, D. Saunders, and G. Khushf. 1998. "An Ethics Discussion Series for Hospital Administrators." *Healthcare Ethics Committee Forum* 10 (20).

Cassidy, J. 1998. "Calvary Hospital Focuses on Ethics." *Health Progress* 79 (6): 48–50, 52.

Ehlen, K., and G. Sprenger. 1998. "Ethics and Decision Making in Healthcare." *Journal of Healthcare Management* 43 (3): 219–221.

Freed, D. 1992. "The Long Distance Administrator." *Health Management Quarterly* 14 (4): 17–20.

Giblin, M., and M. Meaney. 1998. "Corporate Compliance Is not Enough." *Health Progress* 79 (5): 30–31.

Goodstein, J., and B. Carney. 1999. "Actively Engaging Organizational Ethics in Healthcare: Four Essential Elements." *Journal of Clinical Ethics* 10 (3): 224–229.

Goodstein, J., and R. L. Potter. 1999. "Beyond Financial Incentives: Organizational Ethics and Organizational Integrity." *Healthcare Ethics Committee Forum* 11 (4): 288–292.

Hall, R. 1999. "Confidentiality as an Organizational Ethics Issue." *Journal of Clinical Ethics* 10 (3): 230–236.

Heller, J. 1999. "Framing Healthcare Compliance in Ethical Terms: A Taxonomy of Moral Choices." *Healthcare Ethics Committee Forum* 11 (4): 345–357.

Hofmann, P. 1996a. "Achieving Ethical Behavior in Healthcare: Rhetoric Still Reigns Over Reality." *Frontiers of Health Service Management* 13 (2): 37–39.

———. 1996b. "Hospital Mergers and Acquisitions: A New Catalyst for Examining Organizational Ethics." *Bioethics Forum* 13 (2): 45–48.

———. 1998. "Ethics and the CEO (case commentary)." *Hospitals & Health Networks* 72 (2): 32–34.

Johnson, K., and K. Roebuck-Colgan. 1999. "Organizational Ethics and Sentinel Events: Doing the Right Thing When the Worst Thing Happens." *Journal of Clinical Ethics* 10 (3): 237–241.

Joint Commission on Accreditation of Healthcare Organizations. 1998. "Ethical Issues and Patient Rights Across the Continuum of Care." Oakbrook Terrace, IL: JCAHO.

Kalb, P. 1999. "Health Care Fraud and Abuse." *Journal of the American Medical Association* 282 (12): 1163–1168.

Labb, D. 1999. "Defining Appropriate Care: A Matter of Perspective." *Healthcare Executive* 14 (5): 12–16.

Larson, L. 1999. "The Right Thing To Do." *Trustee* 52 (9): 8–12.

Levey, S., and J. Hill. 1986. "Between Survival and Social Responsibility: In Search of an Ethical Balance." *Journal of Health Administration Education* 4 (2): 225–231.

Midgley, M. 1993. "Must Good Causes Compete?" *Cambridge Quarterly of Healthcare Ethics* 2 (2): 131–139.

Nash, L. 1990. *Good Intentions Aside: A Manager's Guide to Resolving Ethical Problems.* Boston: Harvard Business School Press.

Olson, R. 1999. "The Postmodern Prescription: An Antidote to Hard Boundaries and Closed Systems in Healthcare Organizations." *Journal of Clinical Ethics* 10 (3): 178–186.

Ray, L., J. Goodstein, and M. Garland. 1999. "Linking Professional and Economic Values in Healthcare Organizations." *Journal of Clinical Ethics* 10 (3): 216–223.

Rovner, J. 1998. "Organizational Ethics: It's Your Move." *Health System Leader* 5 (1): 4–12.

Rudnick, J. D., Jr. 1995. "Hospital Layoffs: One Facility's Experience with a Work Force Reduction." *Health Progress* (September–October).

Schyve, P. 1996. "Patient Rights and Organization Ethics: The Joint Commission Perspective." *Bioethics Forum* 12 (2): 13–20.

Seely, C., and S. Goldberger. 1999. "Integrated Ethics: Synecdoche in Healthcare." *Journal of Clinical Ethics* 10 (3): 202–209.

Spencer, E., and A. Mills. 1999. "Ethics in Healthcare Organizations." *Healthcare Ethics Committee Forum* 11 (4): 345–357.

Ubel, P., and S. Goold. 1997. "Recognizing Bedside Rationing: Clear Cases and Tough Calls." *Annals of Internal Medicine* 125 (1): 74–80.

Weber, L. 1997. "Taking on Organizational Ethics." *Health Progress* 78 (3): 20.

Worthley, J. A. 1999. *Organization Ethics in the Compliance Context: A Healthcare Management Challenge.* Chicago: Health Administration Press.

Mission and Code of Ethics

Arbuckle, G. 1999. "Mission and Business: Resolving the Tension." *Health Progress* 80 (5): 22–24, 28.

Bianco, D. 1998. "Considering Conversion?" *Trustee* 51 (10): 16–20.

Carlson, G. 1998. "Mission Possible." *Healthcare Executive* 13 (2): 52–53.

Higgins, W. 2000. "Ethical Guidance in the Era of Managed Care: An Analysis of the American College of Healthcare Executives' Code of Ethics." *Journal of Healthcare Executives* 45 (1): 32–42.

Rocky Mountain Center for Healthcare Ethics. 1998. *Colorado Code of Ethics for Healthcare.* Denver, CO: Rocky Mountain Center for Healthcare Ethics.

Tavistock Group. 1999. "A Shared Statement of Ethical Principles for Those Who Shape and Give Health Care." *Annals of Internal Medicine* 130 (2): 144–147.

Tuohey, J. 1998. "Covenant Model of Corporate Compliance." *Health Progress* 79 (4): 70–75.

About the Authors

Paul B. Hofmann, Dr.P.H., FACHE, is vice president of Provenance Health Partners in Moraga, California. In the past, he has been the executive vice president and chief operating officer of the Alta Bates Corporation, executive director of Emory University Hospital, and director of Stanford University Hospital and Clinics. He has also served as Distinguished Visiting Scholar at Stanford University's Center for Biomedical Ethics.

Dr. Hofmann is a fellow of the American College of Healthcare Executives, is a member of ACHE's Leadership Advisory Committee, and is ACHE's consultant on healthcare management ethics and coordinator of its annual ethics conference. He served as chairman of the American Hospital Association's Special Committee on Biomedical Ethics.

Aside from co-editing this book, Dr. Hofmann is the author of over 100 magazine and journal articles. He has held faculty appointments at Harvard, UCLA, Stanford, Emory, and the University of California, Berkeley. He earned his undergraduate, master's, and doctor of public health degrees from the University of California, Berkeley.

William A. Nelson, Ph.D., is an adjunct associate professor of Psychiatry (ethics) and Community and Family Medicine (ethics) at Dartmouth Medical School and the Department of Psychiatry

267

at New York University School of Medicine. In addition, he is the education coordinator for Veterans Health Administration's National Center for Ethics. He has served as co-director of the VA's New England Regional Ethics Center and chief of the Chaplain Service VA Medical Center in White River Junction, Vermont. In 1984, he received the United States Congressional Excalibur Award for Public Service for his work concerning ethical care of the terminally ill. From 1986–1989, he was a W. K. Kellogg Leadership Fellow, studying national and international healthcare policy.

Aside from his role as co-editor of this book, Dr. Nelson is the author of numerous articles and book chapters. He has delivered hundreds of lectures, workshops, and seminars on various healthcare ethics topics. He completed his BA at Elmhurst College; received a M.Div. degree from Andover Newton Theological School; and earned his Ph.D., with a concentration in psychology and ethics, from the Union Institute.

William P. Brandon, Ph.D., MPH, is the Metrolina Medical Foundation Distinguished Professor of Public Policy on Health at the University of North Carolina at Charlotte.

Lawrence B. Chonko, Ph.D., is Holloway Professor of Marketing at Baylor University.

Michael G. Daigneault, Esq., is president of the Ethics Resource Center.

Thomas C. Dolan, Ph.D., FACHE, CAE, is president and CEO of the American College of Healthcare Executives.

Joan Elise Dubinsky, Esq., is president of the Rosentreter Group. She also serves as associate director for employee development at the Howard Hughes Medical Institute.

Gary Edwards, J.D., is president of Meritas Consulting, Inc.

Jane Fulton, Ph.D., is director of School of Natural and Health Science at Barry University.

Susan Dorr Goold, M.D., is director of Bioethics Program at the University of Michigan Medical School. She is also an assistant professor of internal medicine.

John R. Griffith, FACHE, is Andrew Pattullo Collegiate Professor at the School of Public Health, Department of Health Management and Policy, University of Michigan, Ann Arbor.

Marc D. Hiller, Dr.P.H., is associate professor of Health Management and Policy and faculty fellow, Office of the Vice President for Research and Public Service, University of New Hampshire, Durham.

Sister Irene Kraus, LFACHE. We regret that Sister Irene passed away before the publication of this book.

E. Haavi Morreim, Ph.D., is professor at the College of Medicine, University of Tennessee, Memphis.

Laurence J. O'Connell, Ph.D., S.T.D., is the president and CEO of The Park Ridge Center.

David L. Perry is a lecturer at Seattle University's Albers School of Business and Economics–Management.

Frankie Perry, FACHE, retired from her executive vice president position at the American College of Healthcare Executive in 1995. She now serves as an officer in the New Mexico Healthcare Manager's

Forum and edits the newsletter for the University of New Mexico's MPH program.

Edward Petry, Ph.D., is executive director of the Ethics Officer Association.

David C. Thomasma, Ph.D., is the Fr. Michael I. English Professor of Medical Ethics and director of the Medical Humanities Program at Loyola University Medical Center.

Robert E. Toomey, LL.D., LFACHE, is president of Toomey Consulting Services.

Mark H. Waymack, Ph.D., is co-director of Graduate Programs in Health Care Ethics at Loyola University Chicago.

Liz Whitley, Ph.D., and Gerry Heeley, S.T.D., were ethics consultants at Rocky Mountain Center for Healthcare Ethics.

John Abbott Worthley, D.P.A., holds professorships in the United States and Asia. He has been an ethics lecturer around the world and was a principal ethics consultant for the state government of New York.